DOES THIS CLUTTER MAKE MY BUTT LOOK FAT?

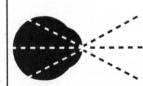

This Large Print Book carries the
Seal of Approval of N.A.V.H.

DOES THIS CLUTTER MAKE MY BUTT LOOK FAT?

AN EASY PLAN FOR LOSING WEIGHT AND LIVING MORE

PETER WALSH

THORNDIKE PRESS
A part of Gale, Cengage Learning

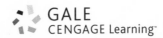
GALE
CENGAGE Learning

Detroit • New York • San Francisco • New Haven, Conn • Waterville, Maine • London

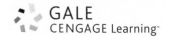
GALE
CENGAGE Learning

Copyright © 2008 by Peter Walsh Design, Inc.

Thorndike Press, a part of Gale, Cengage Learning.

ALL RIGHTS RESERVED

Thorndike Press® Large Print Health, Home & Learning.

The text of this Large Print edition is unabridged.

Other aspects of the book may vary from the original edition.

Set in 16 pt. Plantin.

Printed on permanent paper.

LIBRARY OF CONGRESS CATALOGING-IN-PUBLICATION DATA

Walsh, Peter, 1956–
    Does this clutter make my butt look fat? : an easy plan for los-
ing weight and living more / by Peter Walsh. — Large print ed.
        p. cm.
    Originally published: New York : Free Press, 2008.
    ISBN-13: 978-1-4104-1051-1 (hardcover : alk. paper)
    ISBN-10: 1-4104-1051-X (hardcover : alk. paper)
    1. Weight loss. 2. Consumers. 3. Home economics. 4. Orderli-
ness. I. Title.
    RM222.2.W264 2008b
    613.2'5—dc22
                                                        2008028177

Published in 2008 by arrangement with Free Press, a division of Simon &
Schuster, Inc.

Printed in the United States of America
1 2 3 4 5 6 7 12 11 10 09 08

To the memory of
James Patrick Walsh
1919–2007
My Dad — never afraid to let you know
if your butt was too fat

CONTENTS

INTRODUCTION:
THE EXTRA WEIGHT

A CULTURE OF FAT

The easiest thing to be in America is fat. It's easier than working, easier than raising a family, easier than making money, and definitely easier than getting up and switching off the TV. Being fat has become the national pastime.

When it comes to body size and image, we live in a confused and contradictory world. For all the concern the social commentators, the psychologists, and the politically correct have about the unhealthy influence of those slick fashion and celebrity magazines featuring too-thin models and rapidly reducing stars, that's not where the real problem lies. Yes, the culture of thin that appears in magazines, in movies, and on television is ubiquitous, selling everything from cars to new dentures. But thin's not the story on the street.

The reality is that we worship large. Our

11

cars are the biggest and the fattest — we drive vehicles that consume a gallon of gas every ten miles. Our houses are huge — the average home size is steadily increasing while the average family size is decreasing. Our homes are overflowing with the fat of the things we consume — we spend more time shopping than any other people on earth. Our meals are gargantuan — portion sizes have tripled in the United States over the last twenty-five years. Boeing has increased the assumed weight for each passenger by more than twenty pounds. Office chairs are being made larger to accommodate our bigger butts. Even Disneyland, the happiest — but obviously not the thinnest — place on earth, is redesigning some of its costumes and uniforms to accommodate ever-increasing waist sizes. You'll be happy to know that even if you have a fifty-eight-inch waist and want to work at Disneyland, they have a pair of pants for you! Everywhere we see the effects of an increasingly heavy population — from office chairs to bra sizes, everything is getting bigger. And, most noticeable of all, our pants no longer fit most of us — no surprise since the average waist size has grown four inches in less than ten years. With two-thirds of Americans overweight or obese, it's impossible to deny that we love,

love, love fat.

As a nation we are reveling in an orgy of consumption and it shows no sign of letting up. We can't get enough of anything. The American mantra has become "more is better" and we are applying that motto with gusto to almost every aspect of our lives. If consuming is good, then consuming more is better.

When did buying stuff become a national obsession? When did we become such crazy consumers? When did we get so fat? It all seems to have happened quickly and with little warning. Yesterday you had no trouble fitting into your jeans and today you feel like you're being strangled — at the waistline. America and the world have changed dramatically in our own lifetime. Everything moves more quickly — fast travel, fast mail, fast food. We are all drawn into this ever-quickening pace. "I want it and I want it now" seems almost reasonable. If others can have it, why can't I?

Amazingly, we *have* come close to achieving instant gratification. The 1.3 billion credit cards in circulation in America are one indication that we can buy things the moment the urge strikes us, whether we can afford them or not. We can pay for it later. And plenty of stuff is cheap anyway. We buy

things with little thought of the consequences and, even when buried in debt, our
purchases continue. We can afford a lot and
get it fast. So what do we do? We fill our
houses and our lives with it.

Similarly, food is cheap and immediately
available. We now buy half the food we consume outside our homes. Takeout is quick,
efficient, and cheap. It suits our fast-paced
lives. You don't have to think about what
you're eating — or how much. You'll deal
with it later. Or not. We seem to be genuinely
unaware of the connection between what we
put into our mouths and the size of our
waists. We can even ignore reality by pur-
chasing one of the new digital cameras with
a "slim down" function. Hewlett-Packard's
website promises "the slimming feature,
available on select HP digital camera models, is a subtle effect that can instantly trim
off pounds from the subjects in your photos!" Now you can go down in skinny history. But in the here and now, this convenience comes at a cost. Pig out today, but
strip down to your underwear tomorrow,
stand in front of a mirror, and you'll see the
cost I'm talking about!

When it comes to losing weight, we are
promised the same instant weight loss that
those digital cameras offer. A house can be

14

built on television in a week. An ugly duckling can get a new face and a new body in a mere sixty minutes on prime time. A celebrity can lose the baby weight in three weeks. Who can blame us for expecting the instant fix? But it's all an illusion. Paying with a credit card seems painless, but we all know the bill comes later and has to be paid off with hours of hard work. The same is true when you overeat on a regular basis. Only hard work will get rid of the excess. Our choices today have consequences we have to deal with tomorrow — there's no way around it.

IT'S ALL TOO MUCH:
LIVING A RICHER LIFE WITH LESS STUFF

Four years ago I became the organizational expert on a television show called *Clean Sweep.* The premise of the show was very simple. A team of experts — including me, a designer, a carpenter, and a crew that assisted in the painting and redesign plans — was given two days to help a family dig out from under their overwhelming clutter.

In two days, with a budget of two thousand dollars, we tackled two rooms and really managed to work some miracles. These were not homes with a little clutter here and there. I vividly remember walking into a home where the homeowner said, without flinching, while standing in three-foot-deep clutter, "There is a piano in there somewhere, but I haven't seen it in seventeen years." We found a dining room where the family had not seen the surface of the dining table — much less managed to eat there — for more than six years. And then there was the guy with more than three hundred pairs of shoes — and that wasn't counting what he'd hidden in the garage before I got there! This was clutter that had a life of its own, taking over whole homes and suffocating any chance that the family might have had to live an organized, stress-free life.

The people on *Clean Sweep* may be extreme cases, but this situation is far more common than any of the *Clean Sweep* team had expected. It was not unusual for our production office to receive two hundred and fifty applications *a day,* all begging to be on the show. Like the clutter we saw every day, we were inundated with people needing our help. The sheer weight and volume of what people own is truly overwhelming many homes across America. It's hard to find a home today that has a garage in which there's room left to park a car. There are the houses so full of "stuff" that families are reduced to navigating narrow paths through their clutter. We saw spaces so full of collectibles, furniture, paper, clothes, books, and shoes that even the homeowners themselves seemed mystified by what their lives had become.

What started out as a program to help people deal with clutter quickly morphed into something very different. It became obvious that the clutter represented something much deeper going on in many of the people's lives and relationships. For those people, and many of the clients I work with, a shift had taken place — almost without them realizing it. They no longer owned their stuff; their stuff owned them. For some, it went even further. Their "stuff" was the way they defined themselves — "I am what I own." They were unable or unwilling to separate themselves from what they owned to the point that their living spaces became partially — or in some cases totally — unusable. To break this pattern is an intense challenge. It's not just about putting things in garbage bags or finding the right photo boxes. I help people confront and redefine their relationships with what they own.

The letters that appear throughout this book are a sampling of the many e-mails and notes I receive almost every day. I've removed names and/or stripped away identifying details, but the sentiments are genuine and the people who have expressed them are real.

> Dear Peter:
> I believe that if I can learn to "let go," change will happen. All of this clutter is taking my life away from me. There is so much going on, literally and figuratively, in my house that there is no room for happiness. I find that my body is overwhelmed, my house is overwhelmed, and my mind is overwhelmed. This is a self-imposed prison that I can't get out of. The "clutter" rules every corner of my life.

Each of us has one life. You. Me. Our friends and family. But I have to ask: Is it the life you want? It may be unexpected, but this is the question I always start with when helping people declutter and organize their homes — and ultimately their lives. What is the vision you have of the life you want to live? *Are you living the life you want?*

This is where many of my clients have lost their way. Somehow they've lost sight of what it is they want from the life they have. Almost imperceptibly their stuff infiltrates.

Eventually the clutter fills their space and their life. A sense of frustration and impotence takes over and they feel powerless to turn things around.

Creating a vision for the life you want to live forces you to make decisions based on the real priorities that should drive your life. Do you want to keep the last three years of magazine subscriptions, or do you want to use that dining table for dinner with your family? Do you want to fill the garage with boxes containing your grandmother's moth-eaten tablecloths, or do you want to preserve your investment in your car? Do you want your children's laundry piled on your bed, or do you want your bedroom to be a place of peace and intimacy? Your home shouldn't overwhelm you. It should give you shelter from the storm. And it should be more than a roof over your head. It's up to you to make your home support you in your quest for happiness.

The transformations I have seen are speedy and amazing. As soon as people have space to breathe, their spirits lift. They have new energy and hope. At the end of the process, almost without exception, people tell me, "This has changed my life." Those are amazing and gratifying words to hear. By helping my readers and viewers and clients redefine their relationships to what they own, I have some small part in helping them look differently at their lives. Not in a superficial way, but at a level that has altered their relationships with everyone and to everything around them.

With all my work decluttering homes and watching the resulting transformations came two critical revelations:

1. It's Not About the Stuff

The first step in helping people deal with clutter is to get them to look at things other than the clutter itself. I know this sounds strange, but if you are struggling with the things you own, and focus exclusively on these things, you will never tame them. Believe me, *it's rarely about "the stuff."* Clutter is about fear of losing memories, or worry about the future, or a sense that something bad is going to happen. It's a way of dealing with loss, or even a way of masking the pain of some past trauma. The woman who couldn't let go of family memorabilia because of the sudden and tragic death of her brother, the father who hoarded all of his children's schoolwork because it represented what he felt were the years he was closest to his sons and daughter, or the couple whose home was overflowing with personal paperwork because they were so fearful of identity theft.

Looking beyond the clutter for answers means addressing the underlying issues. I learned long ago that if you focus on the stuff, you will *never* conquer the clutter and deal with the fat and excess that fills your home. This revelation is the key to the success I've had in helping people reframe the way they look at what they own. It is fundamental to helping people overcome years of clutter and disorganization in their lives.

2. Your Home Reflects Your Life

Your home is a reflection of you. Not in some airy-fairy way, but in a real and tangible sense. It's no accident that at the same time we are struggling with the national "epidemic of obesity," we are also living in homes weighted down with clutter and filled with "stuff."

Dealing with clutter and regaining a sense of harmony and organization in their homes touched many people I worked with in ways that I don't think anyone foresaw. Suddenly "clutter" meant so much more than an overstuffed closet or garage. For most, changing their relationship to their stuff became the first step in a larger process of adjusting the other relationships in their lives. Couples reassessed their relationships and removed the hurdles that had cluttered up their emotional lives. A few couples went their separate ways. Others realized that major changes were needed if the relationships were to continue. People lost weight, changed careers, reassessed the way they spent their time, and reorganized their priorities. Removing the clutter from people's lives was more than just clearing a desk of unwanted paperwork or getting all that junk out of the garage. Decluttering and organizing had an impact on every aspect of the lives of the people I worked with.

CLUTTER AND FAT — THEY'RE NOT SO DIFFERENT

Now I want to work with you on a different relationship, another relationship that we lose track of when we're overwhelmed by the pressures and demands of busy lives. Another relationship that is intense, even potentially life threatening, and, when redefined, has the power to change your life. This is a book about you and your relationship with your body — about what you think about it, what you put into it, how you treat it, and whether you are happy with it. In our culture, the relationship most people have with their bodies hinges on size. The size of your body is probably why you picked up this book. And the size of your body is where my expertise as a declutterer comes in. This is a book about the clutter around you and the clutter inside you that prevents you from living the life you want and being the person you wish to be. Your relationship to food is complex. If you're fat, your problems are real, and there are no miracles. Changing is going to take some straight talk and I'm here to give it.

The person for whom clutter is not a problem is extremely rare. So many of my clients seem to have lost focus in their lives and live with a nagging but poorly defined yearning for something they can't quite grasp. In accumulating more and more stuff or eating more and more food, they are attempting to meet the need for "something more." No matter how much more they accumulate, however, the need remains. For others, there is an element of boredom combined with a simmering sense of frustration, even anger. Again, it's something that many find hard to put a finger on, yet whatever it is lies behind their need to fill their lives with things. The hope is that material things will bring meaning and fulfillment. It never works.

All of us deal constantly with the urge to consume more. They're just not very different — clutter and fat: I see it. I want it. I'll have it. Consumption is king. We spend too much, we buy too much, and we eat too much. In the same way that we surround ourselves with so much clutter, we overwhelm our bodies with caloric clutter consisting mainly of sugar and fat. Almost all of us are carrying extra pounds that we just can't seem to shake. The stuff in our homes becomes too overwhelming to deal with, but we keep shopping. Similarly, the increasing weight of our bodies becomes more than we are able to handle, but we keep indulging. I'm not saying that if you're struggling with clutter you'll be fat or that a weight problem automatically means there is clutter in your home. It's not that simple. What is clear, however, is that we have a weight problem in this country and it is killing us. Look around — in all of those fat houses, fat malls, and fat cars are fat people. Clutter and fat — one is a reflection of the other. If you hope to deal with either, you need to change the way you look at things.

It's Not About the Food

As I learned in cluttered houses across the country, when you've collected too much of anything, including fat, you can't get rid of it without facing the underlying issues. To lose weight, to achieve the body and look you desire, you have to consider the many aspects of where and how you live. You have to consider the life you want to live. You have to look at your body the way you look at your house and say, "Do I honor and respect this body? Does it reflect who I am?" If your goals aren't clear and your thinking isn't focused, you can't break the habits that stand in your way.

To deal with the fat that clings to your hips, you need to look beyond the number on the scale. If that's your focus, you will never lose weight. I know that this flies in the face of common thinking, but consider this: Every year, we spend nearly 40 billion dollars on diet books and programs. It's estimated that 45 million of us diet at some point every year and yet we keep gaining weight. If diets are the key to losing weight, why is that with the increasing number of diet books the pounds just keep stacking on? Why, if so many of us diet at least once every year, are two-thirds of us heavier than we should be? As far as I'm concerned, most of those diet books are full of empty promises and short-lived results. They encourage us to spend hours weighing, measuring, and scoring what we put in our mouths. They fill us with a sense of failure and guilt. And each diet book contributes one more piece of clutter to our homes, adding to our already increasing weight — both on our book-shelves and on our hips! More diet books, more weight — a paradox.

The connection between clutter and weight didn't occur to me overnight. About a year ago I published my book *It's All Too Much: An Easy Plan for Living a Richer Life with Less Stuff.* Soon after the book was re-leased I began hearing from people who'd used it to get rid of the clutter in their homes and lives. In these letters I discovered an un-expected side effect. The link that I had sus-pected but only dimly glimpsed became ob-vious through the experiences of my readers. I was inundated with real examples of the impact clutter had on all areas of one's life — especially weight.

Dear Peter:

I have been overweight for most of my adult life. I think about it every day. It is a burden. I've lost the weight and gained it back over and over. I've been around the block long enough to know that I eat to fill a void. What I didn't know was that I was keeping clutter, boxes, and memories in

---

my life for the same reason. Furthermore, the clutter had an invisible hold on me . . . like my weight, my stuff was a burden. And how did I deal with the burden? By eating, of course!

Recently, I read *It's All Too Much* about decluttering my life. I thought I was going to find out how to get rid of some boxes in my basement and, finally, do something with the coconut that my sister sent me forty years ago! What I found was something quite different. In the book you gave me permission to live the life I have always thought about. No, deeper than that, the life I knew I should be living.

After reading your book, I got started on the boxes, the closet, and the garage. I started to feel lighter. Literally. I didn't make the connection to my eating habits and, ultimately, my weight for a couple of weeks. But as I kept working on unloading the clutter of my life, I noticed that I was making better food choices. I wasn't filling up every opportunity with a snack. My desire to work out had come back. I know it sounds strange but it's true. . . . This book clicked on a light that I have been trying to get to for years.

I will never go back because I know that — as you say — it's not about the stuff. And it's not about the weight. It's about my life.

Dozens of my readers started talking to me in letters, at readings, and on the radio. They told me that when they focused on the lives they wanted to live, they were able to free themselves of years of stuff. When they focused on the lives they knew they deserved, they were able to free themselves from years of gorging themselves. And you can, too.

Dear Peter:
I have tried most diets and I have invested in many forms of organizational products and books. Anything that appeared to be "the answer" or "magic bullet" on either front, I was all over it. What I came to discover is that my weight and my clutter have very little to do with food or things and everything to do with my outlook on life. . . . Now that I have gotten rid of a lot of the stuff in my home (I'm just about to do a second round of "the

purge") that made me feel bad, new stuff that I like has appeared. I have also lost ten pounds. The first of many that I need to lose, but I am confident that if I live in the now — by keeping only what I need and love and eating mindfully — I can have the life I was meant to live.

Dear Peter:

I don't find that decluttering my house affects my weight, but I do find that living in a cluttered environment evokes the same feelings as my weight problem. I get the same frustrations — and feelings of utter helplessness — at what feels like an insurmountable problem in both instances. I am using the techniques I learned from *Clean Sweep* and your book to work through my physical clutter, and the feelings I get when I walk into my clutter-free areas are hard to describe. I find myself walking in the rooms and just standing there, looking around.

The feelings of not knowing where or how to start do apply to weight loss, but unfortunately I haven't been able to quite get a handle on the weight side of the equation. I think until I am better able to handle my frustrations with my life and especially my job, I'm just going to have to focus on getting my physical clutter in order, and save the "internal" clutter for another time.

Clutter or weight? Weight or clutter? What is the solution? We have to take a step back and look at the total picture. It's a huge mistake to draw arbitrary lines and to put different parts of your life into separate little boxes. Your food. Your career. Your relationships. Your schedule. Your buying habits. Your diet. Consider for a moment that where you live, what you own, how you interact with others, what you eat, and how you spend your time are all intimately linked. You can't change one piece without affecting all the others.

Dear Peter:
My oldest sister falls into the category of having both a clutter problem and a weight problem. She was chubby as a child and did some yo-yo dieting in her late teens

and twenties. After she married and had her son (and subsequently divorced) she gained a lot of weight. During this time, her home also became a complete nightmare. If I were to take a stab at the cause of both, I would have to say that because she was in an unhappy marriage, she medicated herself with both food and shopping. The weight gain was cyclical, as was the shopping. The more she shopped, the more junk she had around the house, and she got to a point where she just didn't know where to begin. Books and junk everywhere, empty boxes, stuff her ex-husband left (ten years ago) which she's never disposed of. I think that when a person's life is in chaos, that chaos is reflected in all areas of his/her life.

Declutter your mind, declutter your home, declutter your relationship to food. Then watch the ripple effect this has on every aspect of the way you live. Clear out the junk, and in doing so clear out the patterns of thought and behavior that prevent you from living the life you want. If you try to clear the clutter by focusing on the stuff, you will fail to get organized. It's not about the stuff. If you try to lose weight by focusing on the food, you'll never change your body for good. It's not about the food. First define the life you want to live. Acknowledge the issues that clutter that vision. Clean up your priorities. Create a world where those priorities can thrive. Learn how to honor and respect yourself. When you do, the ability to take control of your body will follow.

PERMISSION TO BE IMPERFECT

Thin is not the answer to life's problems. And fat is not life's problem. The focus of my work is to help people be honest with themselves — that's where change starts. Are you stuck in the notion that being ten pounds overweight is wrong and life destroying? Because it's not. Not unless you make it so. And particularly not if you're a sixty-year-old grandparent with a nice, soft lap that's perfect for cuddling the grandkids. Why are some of us perfectionists about weight when we're not perfectionists about anything else in our lives? What is most important to you? It should be personal happiness, love, family, relationships. I'm not in amazing shape myself. I'm over fifty years old, and I'm comfortable. I love the people in my life. I wake up happy in the morning. Life is good. Happiness is the ideal and should be the focus of your priorities. It's the key to a balanced, healthy life.

When I step into a cluttered home, all of the "stuff" recedes into the background. The person or people who live there become my focus — their dreams, their frustrations, their fears, and their hopes. I don't care what your scale says. I don't care what size you wear. I don't care about your BMI (body mass index). I don't care about anything you've put into your mouth before today. I care about the person I meet. How do you feel? Are you happy and at peace with yourself? Do you have energy and enthusiasm? Are you open to new people and experiences? Do you radiate self-confidence and optimism?

I care about the world where you live. Is it safe and comfortable? Do you look forward to walking through your own front door? Is your home a haven? Does it reflect the life you want to live?

I care about the way you treat your body. Do you respect it? Do you get pleasure from physical activity? Do you have a good sex life? Do you sleep well? Are you healthy? Do you enjoy convivial meals with good friends and/or family? Do you have every reason to expect that you'll live long and well?

I want you to live the best life that you can. And I want *you* to decide what that is. I'm not going to tell you to exercise for twenty minutes three times a week. I have no idea if that will make you happy. You need to look to yourself for answers. I'm here to help you do that.

If you're fat and happy, congratulations. You don't need this book. I encourage you to accept yourself as you are. Imperfection is not a problem — unhappiness is. Happiness is the goal here, and a long life in which to enjoy that happiness. If you are fine with your weight and satisfied with your life expectancy, great! You can put down this book, pick up your 750-calorie (not that I'm counting) Starbucks Venti Strawberries & Crème Frappuccino® Blended Crème with whipped cream and call it a day.

Look at your life. If you and your family don't mind the consequences of your weight or if you have a clean bill of health, maybe you should stop harping about those extra ten pounds and enjoy your life. I don't believe in weight loss for the sake of weight loss. I believe in living a life that makes you happy. However, if your butt looks fat and you don't like it, it's time to get rid of it.

A NEW APPROACH

This is not a diet or exercise book. It doesn't have recipes or exercise routines; there are thousands of those you can easily purchase and probably already have. Understand this very clearly — I am *not* a doctor or a dietitian or an exercise physiologist. There are enough experts already cluttering this space and I do not want to add to the frenzy. I am, however, someone who has worked with hundreds of people to get them to a simpler, richer life, one that is less cluttered and more focused. This book is the product of years of experience and a great dose of common sense. I know how to help people gain control of their lives and get out from under the "fat" of what they own. I have seen this hundreds and hundreds of times with clutter and I believe that what is true for our homes and our stuff is also true for our bodies and our weight. It is the remarkable parallel between the weight of clutter and the ever increasing body weight of Americans that has been the driving force behind this book. A cluttered home can have a hugely negative impact on your life. Being overweight or obese can also have devastating consequences for you, your family, and your life.

Unlike the latest fad diet, I'm not promising instant results. If you're looking for a liposuction kit sandwiched between the covers of a book for the suggested retail price of twenty-two dollars, then you've come to the wrong place. You want a quick fix? I'm not your guy. I want you to have long-term results that improve every aspect of your life and, trust me, that can't and won't happen overnight.

The aim of this book is simple: It will show you how to move closer to the life you should be living. It will help you redefine your relationship with your body just as *It's All Too Much* helps people redefine their relationships with their stuff. Your happiness is the goal. Fat, thin, cluttered, clean — I want you to find the life that makes you happy. The world today is a complicated place. For many it's filled with fear and uncertainty. Your weight is actually something you can control. If it's getting in the way of your happiness, let's take care of it once and for all.

You've probably been on a diet before and you probably failed. That's not surprising. Fat, like clutter, can be overwhelming. Excess is always hard to manage — by its very nature, it makes you feel out of control. I'm going to provide you with a clear and simple plan for dealing with the current wave of consumption that affects us all. *Does This Clutter Make My Butt Look Fat?* will help you examine how your emotions, your home, your kitchen, and your pantry are working for — or against — the life you want for yourself. It will ask you to explore the emotional relationship you have with food and eating. It will focus on your personal habits of buying, eating, and exercising so that you can make informed and empowered choices for yourself. If a healthy diet doesn't fit your lifestyle, well, we'll just have to change your lifestyle.

ACTIVITY

Keep or Toss ideas you have about dieting

Diet books and magazines give us a million little tips and tricks for losing weight. Drink ten glasses of water half an hour before you eat. Carbohydrates are evil. Eat only grapefruit for a week and you'll lose weight. Drink one hundred glasses of water a day and you'll never feel hungry again. Salad dressing is bad for you. Dessert is deadly. Every diet has its own science and research and theories and whatever else backing it up. I don't care. It's all clutter. I want you to let go of it. I want you to throw out all the rules you've made for yourself just as surely as later I'm going to ask you to throw out all the bad habits you've accumulated. Of course if something works for you, if you enjoy it, keep doing it. You have room for it in your life. But throw out those weight-loss tricks and ideas that you still hope will be short-cuts to a magical weight loss that takes no work. No more gimmicks.

I'm not here to tell you about food. Chances are you already know more than enough. Fat people know everything there is to know about food: calories, sugar content, nutritional value. You can have a very intimate relationship with food, but don't expect it to be fulfilling. Food, like clutter, promises everything but delivers nothing. This book is not focused on the food you eat, it's about the life you live and how both are deeply linked. Ultimately, it will help you redefine your relationship to what you own, what you eat, and how you live. In so doing, it will change how you live your life.

If you have struggled with the fat that hounds most of us, then here is a chance to look at it in a totally new way. If diet and exercise books have proven useless to you, if you yearn to make a change but don't quite know how, then it's time to make a change that works.

I'm not saying it will be easy or the results immediate, but I have helped people across the country deal with the excess of clutter that has robbed them of pleasure and enjoyment. Together, we can apply those same lessons to the stretch-elastic waistbands that haunt us every day! I promise that if you embrace *Does This Clutter Make My Butt Look Fat?* you will come away with strategies and techniques to make lasting changes in your life.

You hold the solution in your hands. The choice is yours.

ONE:
THE LIFE YOU HAVE

HOW HEAVY IS THE WEIGHT YOU BEAR?
Did you know that researchers have estimated that by 2015, three-quarters of the
population in this country will be obese or
overweight? That's more than 225 million fat
people! With all that company, what's so bad
about fat? Is your fat harmless? Or does it
permeate all aspects of your health and happiness? Use this quiz to evaluate how much
it plays in to different aspects of your life.

QUIZ

The Weight of Weight

1. How is your physical health?
   a. I have energy most days and gen-
      erally feel fine. My doctor says I
      could lose a few pounds.
   b. I have my ups and downs but I get
      by.

   c. I have some health problems. Who doesn't?

2. If a social group that you belong to organized a softball game, how would you participate?
   a. I'd play till the bitter end, no matter how far in outfield they made me stand.
   b. I'd volunteer to restock the cooler.
   c. I'd stay home. Nobody needs a permanent mental image of my ass sliding into home base.

3. If you won an all-expenses-paid beach retreat, would you go?
   a. I'd hop on the first plane.
   b. I'd go and have a great time, even if I were hidden in a coverup, forbidding any photos to be taken.
   c. I'd trade in my prize for cash dollars. Nobody's seeing me in a bathing suit.

4. When you last tried something new (taking a dance class, putting together a piece of furniture, doing a home re-

pair, driving an unfamiliar rental car), how would you describe your ability to get the hang of it?

a. I'm not superfast or talented, but I get by just fine.

b. I tend to be a little clumsy and slow.

c. Dance classes? Home repairs? You gotta be kidding. I don't go near that stuff.

5. Which of the following statements best describes your current or most recent relationship while it was occurring?

a. My partner loves my body and/or is into me for who I am as a person.

b. I always try hard to look good for my partner, but am never quite sure s/he is attracted to me.

c. My partner is critical of my body — even if s/he doesn't say anything, I can tell.

6. When it comes to my family . . .

a. We spend lots of time together doing a variety of activities — a mix of calm and active.

b. I guess we get along. We watch a lot of TV together!

c. I don't always have the energy to be the parent I'd like to be.

7. What best describes your sex life over the past five years?
   a. My sex life is active and fulfilling.
   b. My partner and I don't always see eye-to-eye on how much is enough sex, but it's okay.
   c. What sex life?

8. Do you have the career you'd like to have?
   a. I like my job and the people I work with. No complaints.
   b. This isn't my ideal job, but it pays the bills.
   c. I'm frustrated at work. I try so hard and my efforts go unappreciated. I might even deserve a raise or pro-motion that hasn't been offered.

9. What best describes your attitude at work?
   a. I'm skilled at what I do and confi-

dent in my abilities.

b. The work piles up and it's hard to stay on top of it. It's always on the verge of getting out of control.

c. I'm in way over my head and barely surviving here. I always feel like they're about to fire me, and why shouldn't they? Someone else could do a much better job.

10. How would you describe your personal financial situation?

a. I work; I save; I should be able to retire comfortably at sixty-five.

b. I make ends meet, but I really should be on a tighter budget.

c. I earn a decent living, but I have credit card (or other) debt and can't get out from under it.

11. When I think about the life I'm living . . .

a. I love my friends and family. Life's not perfect, but when I look in the mirror and around my house, I feel happy.

b. Sometimes I can't believe this is the way my life turned out. It's just not what I expected. Of all the lives I could have had . . . I have no idea why I ended up here.

c. I don't like to look in the mirror and be reminded of who I am. My house makes me depressed. I wish it were different but I can't begin to make a change.

SCORE YOURSELF

If your answers were mostly As:

If most of your answers were As, congratulations! You're in good shape. Your weight doesn't weigh heavily on you. You're relatively happy with your body, both how it looks and how it feels. You're open to trying new things. You have good relationships with your family and friends. Your work life is satisfying. The life you have is pretty close to the life you want. Do you really need to lose weight? Or would you do better to free yourself from some contrived ideal? There's nothing wrong with continuing your efforts to live your ideal life. You can use this book to fine-tune. But I want you to make sure to be realistic and to take pleasure in the good life you have.

If your answers were mostly Bs:

You're in the middle ground here — you're not in love with your life, a little confused and unsure, but not miserable. That's a small but troublesome load you're trying to bear. It's hardest to change when you're just managing to get by. You know things could be better, but motivating is easier when you've hit rock bottom. Why wait? Don't settle for an okay life. It's time to make a change.

If your answers were mostly Cs:

Your weight is getting in the way of your life. The areas of life that are most important to you — be they family, relationships, job, or being adventurous and happy with yourself — are suffering. But the good news is that you've already admitted that you know you need a change. Once you focus on what's important and make choices that support your priorities, you'll see that change comes speedily and naturally.

YOU'RE NOT ALONE

There are plenty of statistics circulating about the fattening of America, what is causing it, and the problems it is causing. But statistics don't matter to individuals. Having the "facts" doesn't guarantee better behavior. The solution for *you,* for your weight problem, isn't in statistics or government-recommended diets. It's not in food labels or BMI calculators. The only way to change, and change for good, is for you to take interest in your own body and what you put into it, to be informed, and to take responsibility for the extra fat that weighs you down and impedes your ability to live the life you want. Weight control is not about diets, it's about decisions. Your decisions.

YOU ARE FAT — NO EXCUSES

> Dear Peter:
> What would I do with myself if all these issues were resolved? What would I do if I was at a weight where I just felt comfortable with myself? What would I do if I no longer had to take medication for depression/anxiety? What would I (and my family) do if our house was not wall-to-wall clutter? That's kind of scary to think about — I wouldn't have any excuses anymore. Hmmm . . .

If you have a medical problem, of course you should seek medical help. But do you actually have a medical problem or are you turning to doctors in hope of handing over responsibililty for the problem? Be honest. True, if you're fat, you are definitely on your way to lots of health issues, but long before that happens you still have the power to turn things around. Enough of the excuses already! It's not for me to tell you what life to live. I have no interest in doing that. The road you follow is your choice. But realize that when you make that choice you have to accept the consequences or find another route.

DON'T YOU DARE CALL ME FAT!

Have you wondered yet why I am using the word "fat" instead of the more politically correct "overweight" or "obese"? The reason is that "fat" is simple. It's a strong, straightforward word. "Overweight" and "obese," on the other hand, sound too formal, too medical, too polite. Let's use real words for real problems. For most of us, fat is not a medical problem . . . yet. Of course, there are people for whom excess weight is a medical condition that requires medical intervention. Common sense tells us that. But the same common sense suggests that two-thirds of this country could not, in less than a generation, develop a weight condition that is a medical problem. My point is that the terms "obese" and "overweight" are so polite or medical that they take the burden away from you, and you're the one who ate all that food. The moment your weight is labeled a "medical problem," the only way to solve it is through consultation with an expert, a selection of treatment options, ongoing consultation, probable medication, and the long wait for the much-anticipated cure. This isn't a condemnation of the medical profession. In this country the medical establishment is focused on treatment and when you knock on their door that's what they'll offer — a pill, a referral, or a gastric band. Medicine isn't going to solve your problems. You are. We are fat. Fat. Fat. Fat. The solution you're looking for is a lot closer than a trip to your primary care physician.

Maybe you recognize yourself somewhere here:

I don't have time to do whatever it is you're about to tell me to do.

I've tried dieting and it doesn't work.
I love food and can't stop eating it.
Fat is in my family. It's a genetic thing. I
* can't help it.*
I cheat on diets so they never work.

These are strikingly similar to the excuses I hear about clutter every day. Let me address them one by one.

Excuse # 1: "I don't have time to do whatever it is you're about to tell me to do."

Life is an ongoing balancing act of time and priorities. Our lives are full, and that's a good thing. But I want you to take a moment to think about the time you already spend dealing with your weight.

- Do you spend time feeling guilty about what you've eaten?
- Do you spend time in front of the mirror changing clothes because you don't feel good in anything you own?
- Do you spend time shopping for clothes because it's hard to find clothes that fit well and hide whatever it is you're trying to hide?
- Do you spend hours at the gym trying to burn off the extra dessert you allowed yourself last night?

- Have you tried so many diet books and programs that they're all a blur of protein bars and chemical milkshakes?
- At the rate you're going, will you spend time at the doctor's dealing with the medical conditions your weight will eventually cause?

Think about all the time that your weight consumes. Consider the mental anguish it causes. Imagine being free of that. Imagine being able to throw on anything in your closet knowing it can't look too bad because you're happy with your body and weight. Now tell me you don't have time to invest in feeding your body the healthy food it deserves.

Excuse # 2: "I've tried dieting and it doesn't work."

Agreed. Dieting doesn't work. Have you ever met someone who used to be fat but conquered the problem long ago? That person probably doesn't say, "I've been on a diet for ten years." She says, "I learned how to eat." Think of it this way: If your new eating plan succeeds, it's a change in your life. If it fails, it's a diet.

This is not a diet book and I'm not talking about you going on another diet. Nearly forty-five million Americans diet every year and most of them end up feeling like failures. Worse still, many quickly regain the weight they lost, and then some. Diets are constantly presented as the way to lose weight, but all of our experience tells us that diets simply don't work. Part of the problem is that a diet is something you go "on." If you go "on," then at some point you're going to go "off." You can't clean up the clutter in your house once and expect it to stay clutter-free from then on. We're talking about an ongoing process here, not a one-off event. You can't take some food plan, live by it for a few months until you reach your ideal weight, then go back to eating the same way you always did. Your health is not about having a list of what you can or can't eat. Your health is not an on-or-off proposition. To really change your weight you have to change your total life. You have to change the choices that you make every day — about how you live, how you respond to others, how you feel, what you value, who you love, how you spend your time, and how you interact with the world around you. This is the kind of "balanced diet" that will bring lasting, long-term results. We are going to examine your relationship with food and redefine it in terms of your total life. If you are honest with yourself you can succeed.

Excuse # 3: "I love food and can't stop eating it."

Who says you should stop eating food? On the contrary, I want you to love your food. I want you to enjoy it. And I don't want you to feel bad about it afterward. There is, however, a difference between loving food and out-of-control eating. Part of loving someone is the understanding that you also respect that person. It is no different with the food that you put into your body. Food is essential — without it we simply cannot continue to exist. Respecting and valuing your life means respecting and valuing your body. If you truly love food, then you should have respect for how and what you eat. Is what you love real food, or is it a chemically processed product with lots of salt, sugar, and fat, and little nutritional value? What would happen if you replaced these foodlike products with real food prepared by real people with real love? What would happen if you ate with your friends or family in a place that makes you happy and comfortable? What would happen if you were fully aware of the food you were putting into your body? Let's see what happens then.

Excuse # 4: "Fat is in my family. It's a genetic thing. I can't help it."

What I hear in this excuse is: I'm not the only one who's fat. My whole family has the same problem. It's not my fault, it's in my genes. Oh, and pass me another cookie! I'm not surprised if your whole family has a similar problem but that doesn't automatically make it something in your DNA. Too often the genetic or the medical excuse is used as a get out of jail free card, a way to sidestep personal responsibility. Chances are you all grew up eating the same foods and you probably have the same relationship with food. What I *don't* hear in this excuse is: I eat food that is good for me in reasonable portions. What I don't hear is: If I gave my doctor an honest diary of everything I've eaten in the last month he'd say I have a wonderfully nutritious diet and that my bloodwork reflects that. Of course genes play a role. It may be harder for you to be slender than it is for your size-two nemesis. I don't expect you to work miracles. I want you to live with the confidence that you're being the best you can be.

Excuse # 5: "I cheat on diets so they never work."

Of course you cheat. We all do! But face it, if you cheat on your diet then you are lying to yourself. It's self-destructive behavior and you know it. So the question is, Why are you doing it? What turned you into your own enemy and how can you change? What is causing you to lose control? It's time to think about your food choices differently. You've come to the right place.

FAT GETS IN THE WAY OF LIFE

It's easy to get fat. Easy as pie. And ice cream. And soda. And chips. Easy as super-sized fast food and hundreds of cable channels available at the click of a remote. All you have to do to be fat in this country is go with the flow. Eat what the advertisers want you to eat. Buy what the grocery stores sell you. Finish what the restaurants put on your plate. Do what everyone else does for a decade or so and congratulations! You're fat!

It's easy to get fat. But it's not so easy to *be* fat. Fat isn't just a matter of not liking what you see when you look in the mirror. Remember — all the parts of our lives are interconnected. Is your fat causing any of the problems below? Is fat getting in the way of living the life you want?

Fat comes between you and your relationships

Feeling physically limited handicaps your

ability to be the lover, husband, wife, mother, father, or friend you wish to be. Do you have the energy to do anything and everything you'd like to do with your partner, your children, your grandchildren? Has your weight changed significantly since you and your partner met? Do you still feel as attractive? Are you still attracted to each other or is your fat literally coming between the two of you? I don't like to say that fat is unattractive, and I don't have to. Society says it for me in hundreds of negative and often hurtful ways in ads, on TV, in movies, on billboards, in high school classrooms, in government elections, at water coolers, and on the beach. If you're fat, I'm afraid you're being told in hundreds of subtle and not-so-subtle ways every day. Hearing it from your partner, or would-be partner, does untold damage to your psyche and your relationship. Maybe worse, feeling unhappy with your body isn't good for you or your partner. When my client Heather feels heavy, she insists on having the lights off when she has sex with her husband. Is your partner supposed to treat you with honor and respect when you don't treat yourself that way? Your fat doesn't just interfere with your physical abilities. It bulges out into the most important relationships of your life.

Reality Check

It can be easy to convince yourself that an extra pound here or there isn't noticeable. Try this little exercise. Set up a video camera on a tripod or shelf somewhere private in your home. Set up the camera to tape you from about ten feet away. Strip down to your underwear — or further, if you're really brave — and then do some jumping jacks in front of the camera.

The tape will give you a chance to see how your body moves with the extra weight you are carrying. This isn't intended to humiliate or depress you. It's simply an opportunity to glimpse how you look objectively. Trust me, I've done it myself. It can be a real wake-up call.

Now *destroy the tape!* The Internet can be a dangerous thing!

You can also try this exercise in front of a full-length or three-way mirror. Every night, if that's what it takes. Try promising yourself that before you open the refrigerator you'll do naked jumping jacks. A reality check can be quite an appetite suppressant.

Fat robs you of career opportunities

If you're overweight, don't be surprised if you have trouble landing the job you want. When it comes to being hired and promoted, trim, fit-looking people definitely have the edge over their fat colleagues. Recent research shows that only 9 percent of top male executives are overweight and, amazingly, that overweight people can expect to earn 10 to 20 percent less than their thinner coworkers. Weight discrimination in the workplace is harder to prove and usually couched in subtle but unmistakable terms. Women are particularly hard hit in this area, with one study quoting 60 percent of employers saying that they would either not hire, or only hire under specific circumstances, women who were obese. The stereotype of the fat person is someone who is lethargic, lazy, and has little self-control. This is a huge hurdle for any candidate with weight issues to overcome.

Fat endangers your mental health

The unfortunate truth is that fat people are frequently the butt of mean jokes, negative stereotyping, or derision. It's tough to be the fat kid in school. No one sets up the fat girl in the office on a blind date. People who'd never tell racist or sexist jokes don't think twice about making a fat joke. It's wrong and it's cruel.

Prejudice can very easily push a person into a downward spiral of anger, low self-esteem, hopelessness, and even self-loathing. Hopelessness goes hand-in-hand with help-lessness, and this inevitably leads to seeking comfort in the way we know best — more food. Sometimes the only way out of a vicious cycle is to work on both problems — the clutter and the depression — at the same time.

Dear Peter:

I suffer from depression and have finally gotten treatment in the last year. One thing I've come to realize is how "checked out" of life I had been before. When I look around my home, I see years of neglect, just not being present and taking care of the "stuff" around me. With three kids and a husband, the "stuff" can really pile up if no one is managing it. And I see the same thing with my weight and health. Instead of being present in my life, taking care of myself, eating healthy, etc., I was just existing and eating and not really being aware or taking time for self-care.

> The cluttered home and neglected body are the cause and effect of the depression. Together they form a vicious cycle. Your home is frustrating and overwhelming, your body is frustrating and overwhelming, and it's easy to "check out." Which makes the home even worse, the body get unhealthier, etc., etc.
>
> And as I feel a sense of control over my external environment (my home), it also helps me feel empowered to take better care of my body.

Fat robs you of your physical health

We hear about the health risks associated with being fat all the time. The most common ones are diabetes, heart disease, and stroke, but fat also can cause pregnancy complications, incontinence, herniated or slipped disks, heartburn, arthritis, acid reflux, and even some forms of cancer.

But wait, there's more. Being fat makes it harder to move around, a situation often compounded by damage to joint bones and cartilage. It's highly likely that you'll have more problems getting a good night's sleep because of sleep apnea, snoring, or other breathing complications simply from the pressure on your lungs. It will be tougher to keep up with your children, climb a flight of stairs, or take part in an activity that demands concentrated physical effort. Fat gets in the way of any career that requires you to be active and energetic. You don't need me to tell you any of this. The bottom line is that fat affects your health enormously.

Fat robs you of your quality of life

Fat inhibits you from participating in the pleasures life has to offer. Think about the inhibitions fat creates: Have you ever avoided a swim party or the beach because the idea of shopping for a bathing suit, much less wearing one, was too horrifying? Do you feel comfortable on the dance floor? Fat causes physical discomfort: Are you comfortable in an airplane seat? (Okay, *nobody* is comfortable in an airplane seat, but does your fat make matters worse?) Is it an effort for you to get in and out of the car? When you make plans to go to a restaurant, do you worry about the flimsy-looking chairs?

Fat is bad for the budget

How much does it cost America to have 60 percent of its population overweight? These costs have been estimated to exceed $117 billion every year. That number represents both direct costs — things like increased treatment or more diagnostic tests — and indirect costs — like lost wages because of an inability to work or the amount of earnings lost because of an early death associated with being overweight. Most of these costs stem from the expense associated with diagnosing and treating heart disease, hypertension, and type 2 diabetes.

The United States is losing nearly 40 million workdays a year because of obesity, and we are visiting our doctors 60 million times more than we need to and spending nearly 90 million days confined to bed. With the strain this puts on the medical system, no wonder you have to wait more than a week for a doctor's appointment! All because we are simply too fat.

A recent study suggested that the annual medical costs for an obese person are nearly 40 percent more than those for a person of normal weight. These costs already exceed the health costs associated with smoking.

THE LIFE YOU'RE LIVING IS MAKING YOU FAT

Look, it's not rocket science. If you stand in front of an oncoming bus, you're going to get hurt. If you sit on the sofa in front of the TV every night from 7:30 until the eleven o'clock news, drinking soda and eating takeout, you'll be fat. Period. End of story. I don't want to hear about gland problems, big bones, or inherited fat supercells. Your choices have consequences. There is no magic cure. Food is not some hypnotic, evil force against which we are powerless. Food is delicious. It gives us energy. Eating is joyous. It should give us pleasure, pleasure that we share with our friends and family. I'm not here to provide you with recipes for low-fat chicken and instructions on how to make a salad. You know as well as I do what constitutes a healthy diet: lots of fresh fruit and vegetables, some lean protein, some whole grains. Come on, do you really need me or another diet book to spell it out for you? I don't think so. We know how to eat right, but we don't do it. Why not?

You're victim to the same culture of clutter and excess as the rest of us, but that doesn't let you off the hook. The life you are choosing to live is making you fat. Nobody's forcing those french fries into your mouth. No one's insisting that you clean your plate (or they shouldn't be!). It's time for you to step up, to take control back, to drive your own life. You have the power to make healthy, tasty food decisions. But you've relinquished that power to junk-food manufacturers who've given us all a craving for chemically sweet, nutritionally void snack foods; to a society that considers fat a problem that a doctor should solve; to all the miracle diets that you want to solve your problems instantly and effortlessly. Most of all, you've relinquished power to your own bad habits.

I've talked to countless people who go on and off and on and off diets. They lose the weight they want to lose, live like that for a while, then the weight creeps back on and they go back on the diet. Going on and off diets is about gaining and losing control of what you eat — it's about making and not making the choices that are best for you. Are you really going to be on a diet for the rest of your life? No. Instead, you need to actively make positive choices about what you're going to eat every day until you die. (And, chances are, the more control you have, the longer you'll live.) In the same way that people can conquer the overwhelming weight of stuff in their homes, you can conquer that stubborn extra weight on your hips and butt. It can be done, but you're the one who has to do it.

CLUTTER MAKES YOU FAT, FAT MAKES YOU CLUTTERED

Physical clutter makes you fat

The cookbooks that fill your countertop, leaving you no space to prepare and cook healthy meals, are making you fat.

The thin clothes that you hope will fit again one day are making you fat.

The baggy clothes that you hide behind are making you fat.

The garage full of unused exercise equipment is making you fat.

The boxes of memorabilia that keep you living in another time are making you fat.

The pantry chock full of disorganized food is making you fat.

Even the dining room table covered with mail is making you fat.

I've said it before and I'll say it again: Clutter gets in the way of living the life you want. It makes it hard to breathe. It makes it hard to move. It makes it hard to see clearly. It makes it hard to focus and stay motivated. You have to clean outside to get clean inside.

Collecting clutter is a habit. It may be a passive habit — you let the incoming mail accumulate — nonetheless, it is a pattern you have to break. In *It's All Too Much* I explain how to break this pattern by dealing with the underlying issues as you remove the clutter. But it's a chicken-and-egg situation. You need to clarify your priorities so that you can make choices to get rid of stuff. However, as your space becomes clutter-free and pleasant, it's easier to see your priorities and make the right choices: chicken, egg. I'm here to help you discover the underlying issues at the same time that you clean up your act.

Yes, clutter gets in the way of your relationships, your career, your sense of fulfillment, your happiness. But the connection between physical clutter and weight gain seems to be particularly strong. The more cluttered your space is, the more weight you gain. The fatter you get, the more clutter creeps in. And as you clean up, the weight will fall away. And as the weight falls away, you'll have more energy and will to take control of your space. This is the clutter-weight cycle.

Dear Peter:

When I hold on to clutter, I'm often procrastinating and unmotivated, and therefore not exercising as regularly and likely grazing some snacks in response to viewing the pile of papers on my desk! Then five or ten pounds creep on. I declutter, take charge of my life again, feel more like exercising and less like snacking. . . . Then the weight goes down again. They're long, gradual cycles, like over one to five years. It's simply eating for emotional not physical reasons, as keeping the clutter for me represents emotions and/or thoughts I'm stuck on.

Emotional clutter makes you fat

Just as collecting clutter is tied to underlying issues, you have unhealthy eating habits that are tied to certain emotional triggers: a time or place where you overindulge, an emotion which you feed with food, a need for instant gratification or comfort, a desire to reward yourself for an achievement, a feeling that you deserve a treat after a tough day. You are in the habit of satisfying these emotions by eating things you know are bad for you — or would, if you stopped to think about it. It's the same clutter-weight cycle I see with physical clutter. Acknowledge your emotional clutter and find new ways to deal with it, and the fat will fall away. As the fat disappears, you'll find you have better control of the emotions. But as soon as you let your emotions — be they depression, exhaustion, anger, or joy — make your eating decisions for you, the weight will creep on, and that extra weight will lead to more depression, exhaustion, and anger, and not so much joy. I'm going to show you how to identify your trigger emotions, and how to form new associations so you can break the emotional eating habit.

It's time to sort through these habits and do some personal spring cleaning. And some summer, fall, and winter cleaning. Time to clean up your surroundings and break the habits that steer you in the wrong direction.

Your choices have consequences. Every time you pull out your credit card to buy another pair of shoes or toy or collectible, you're making a choice to bring that item into your home, to add to your clutter problem. Every time you put a bite in your mouth, you are choosing to bring that piece of food into your body, to add to your weight problem. Keep this in mind: Every roll of fat on your body came from something you chose to put into your mouth. And every pound that slips away is going to be because of a decision you make.

One of the greatest lessons I've learned in helping people declutter their lives is that each of us is stronger than we think, and the initial commitment you make is the most difficult step toward change. This is your life. It's the only life you have. If you're not happy and satisfied, that's your problem and you can fix it. I'm just going to break it down into simple steps for you. I'm going to help you see what you want and how to get it. I couldn't count a calorie if my life depended on it. Actually, I probably could, but I'm not going to bother because that's not where the solution lies.

ORGANIZATION FOR HEALTHY LIVING

The move from chaos to calm is not impossible. When it comes to decluttering homes, I find myself telling people the same things over and over again. Common sense and a trust in your "inner voice" should be your guide. The same is true for weight loss.

CLUTTER PRINCIPLES

1. Decluttering your home is the first step toward living your ideal life.
2. Imagine the life you want and hold that idea in your mind as you work through the process.
3. Figure out what your goal is for a room. If an item doesn't serve that goal, get rid of it.
4. If you don't love it, use it, wear it, or have room for it, get rid of it. It's clutter.

5. The clutter didn't appear overnight and won't disappear overnight.
6. Live firmly in the present, not the past or the future. If you're holding on to things you don't use, figure out why. Memory? Hope? Gift? Fear?
7. Break decluttering into small, manageable tasks.
8. If you don't make decluttering a way of life, the stuff will creep back into your home.
9. Decluttering teaches you how to verbalize what's important to you and to make choices based on those priorities.
10. Recognize and celebrate every space that's decluttered. It will motivate you to keep going.

What I tell people is simple: You can't fit five cubic feet of stuff into three cubic feet of space. You only have the space you have. If you only bring things into your home and don't take anything out, sooner or later you will have no room. If you don't use, love, and honor something it has no place in your home. Just because someone gave you something doesn't mean you have to keep it. You must respect the limits of the physical space that you have, because if you don't the space can't function and your vision is lost. None of this is new information and none of what I recommend is magic — it's just good old-fashioned common sense.

You can't lose weight if your home is out of control. If your house isn't welcoming, you won't want to spend time there and you certainly can't expect to enjoy meals there. Just as you must respect the limits of the physical space that you have, you must respect the limits of your body. If you consume an unhealthy quantity of food, your body will cease to look good and perform at its best. Let's look at the same list of clutter principles again, this time substituting weight and weight loss for clutter and decluttering.

FOOD-CLUTTER PRINCIPLES

1. Imagine the life you want and hold that idea in your mind as you work through the process.
2. Organizing where, how, and what you eat is the first step toward achieving your ideal body.
3. Figure out what your goal is for your body. If a food doesn't serve that goal, don't eat it.
4. If it isn't healthy, colorful, and part of your meal plan, don't eat it. It's junk.
5. The fat didn't appear overnight and won't disappear overnight.

6. Live in the present, not the past or the future. If you're eating for emotional reasons, figure out why. Anger? Despair? Comfort? Fear?
7. Focus on enjoying the next meal. Don't let one mistake make you give up.
8. If you don't make mindful eating a way of life, the fat will creep back onto your butt.
9. Taking time to think out your meals teaches you how to verbalize what's important to you and to make choices based on those priorities.
10. Recognize and celebrate every meal you enjoy. It will remind you of the great things a meal provides, beyond just the food.

The math of weight is the same as that of clutter: You can only have as many books as you have room on your shelves or only the number of shirts that can hang comfortably in your closet; if you eat more calories than your body needs, they will be stored as fat. Of all the possessions in your home, your body should be your most treasured. Treating your body with honor and respect means you are treating yourself with honor and respect.

Again, what I am saying is nothing new

and it's not magic, but if you live by these principles, you'll see real changes.

I am not going to tell you, meal by meal, what foods you should and shouldn't put in your body. After all those failed diets, this should be a relief to you. Food is part of the equation — it has to be. So yes, I will ask you to make decisions about what goes into your body. And yes, I will ask you to get rid of some of the food cluttering your pantry. But I'm not going to tell you to eat one-fifth of an egg white at 6:00 a.m. while chugging a protein drink and jumping up and down. Instead, we're going to work on taking control of your life, particularly the part of your life that's related to your weight.

Organization is control, and that is the key to healthy living. Organize your home and you'll stop feeling stressed and over-whelmed. Organize your meals and you won't default to eating takeout or frozen pizza. If you don't make conscious decisions, the world has a way of coming in and making them for you. And the world we live in happens to favor TV, sugar, fat, salt, inactivity, and a myriad of other fat-causing options.

It's time to start making personal choices. Choices that make sense for you. Now, together, we're going to start making decisions again. We're going to take control. We're going to get organized. The process is simple. Here's how it works.

1. The Life You Want

When I help people clean up their houses, we don't start by talking about what to throw away. We talk about what matters. As with your house, so, too, with your body. I'll ask you to think about your life, what it looks like today, and how you want it to be in the future. We'll define the gap between the life you live and the life you want. Redefining yourself and your goals is the first step toward making a fresh start. Instead of picking a weight goal and focusing on the scale, you'll translate your ideal weight into tangible goals — how you want to feel and what you want to do. By doing this, you set yourself on a path that is much more meaningful than some three-digit number on the scale.

2. The Emotions You Confront

We eat because we are human. We need calories to live. To some extent, we overeat because we invented foods with processed sugars and saturated fats in quantities that aren't found in nature. But for most of us there is an emotional component to overeating. We can't summon the strength to make choices about what we put in our bodies. We'll explore these issues and I'll suggest ways you can break emotional habits.

3. The Home Where You Live

Remember the clutter-weight cycle? If your home, where you spend a good portion of your time, is out of control, how can you expect to have control over your food-related decisions? I already wrote an entire book about decluttering your home, but here we'll look specifically at the fat-fueling clutter in your house and clean up your act so you have the space and clarity to redefine your relationship with your body.

4. The Kitchen You Create

It's impossible to cook healthy food and enjoy it if your kitchen isn't a pleasant place to be. I'll walk you through every step of making your kitchen, your pantry, and your refrigerator engines that drive your new life approach.

5. The Food You Stock

Next, we'll learn how to plan. Planning sounds like it involves too many lists and charts, but what planning actually means is figuring out the path toward your goals. Ever used the Web to map a driving route? Then you know that planning saves time. We'll talk about finding time where none seems to exist, planning meals, and how to shop for them.

6. The Meals You Prepare

Eating well isn't just about planning healthy meals. You have to set aside time for those meals. Make them rich and satisfying. Enjoy the ritual of preparing and eating your food, whether you eat alone or with others. If you don't learn to do that, you'll still look for quick satisfaction in easy, empty calories.

7. The Life You Live

Everything is connected. You'll never lose weight if the rest of your life is cluttered, stressful, or unfulfilling. Look at all aspects of your life, particularly your exercise habits, to boost the energy that you have to organize a healthy diet.

8. The Challenges You Face

Even if you manage to cook healthy foods at home, it can all fall apart when you venture out into the real world. We'll identify the high-risk situations that trigger your overeating and consumption of unhealthy food, and I'll give you tactics for how to avoid or overcome temptation.

9. The Success You Enjoy

Finally, we'll talk about success and how to sustain it. This is not a diet. It is a total life approach. If you're going to be a healthy weight for the rest of your life, you're going to have to make permanent changes that support, encourage, and cultivate that weight. We're going to lock them in for good.

CHECKLIST FOR CHAPTER ONE

- ❏ Take the Weight of Weight quiz.
- ❏ Quit making excuses.
- ❏ Reality check — Do jumping jacks in front of a video camera.

Two:
The Life You Want

Choose Your Own Adventure

The only person who can create the life you want is you. Like it or not, no knight in shining armor is coming to make the situation better for you. Your destiny is firmly in your own hands. If you are unhappy with the life you have or unsatisfied with the body you have, then you should change it, and I would like to help you. I want you to live the best life you can. Fat wreaks havoc and it's impossible to ignore. Like clutter, it literally gets in your way. Here's how we clear the path.

This is no ordinary weight-loss program. We don't start with waist measurements, body-fat percentages, or scales. When you focus on the numbers you're trying to fix the wrong problem. Instead, we're going to start with you! Let's sit down, take some time, and think things through. It sounds vague now, but stay with me here. Take the example of one of my readers — let's call her Judy — who lives in an apartment in Falls Church, Virginia. The clutter that filled her apartment always seemed insurmountable. But she had a turning point when she decided to sit down and think through the purpose for each room in her apartment. Thinking about her life, deciding what she wanted, and having a plan helped Judy dive into the work, and it didn't take long for her to see changes.

Dear Peter:

[I] had an "aha" moment when you said, "Decide the purpose of the room first, before you declutter anything." That took the fear and frustration right out of me. I suddenly relaxed and realized I had continually shoved around thirty years of clutter in my apartment and done little else. I laid out what I wanted in each section of my apartment — things like I want my dining room table in front of the patio balcony because I have a lovely view, and my desk and work area back where the dining room used to be.

Friday I cleaned my bathroom and added a new shower curtain, rugs, etc. I also cleaned my kitchen — defrosted and

> emptied the fridge, restored the cabinets and floors, and unpacked china, flatware, and glasses. In two days I did more work on my apartment than I had in decades.

Organizing and decluttering had an immediate side benefit for Judy. After those first two days of cleanup she got on the scale and noticed that she "lost seven pounds in two days." She'd been working so hard and with such focus that she hadn't had time for snacks. But she wasn't counting on short-term results. Her efforts to clean up her house fed directly into her weight-loss goals. Now, because her clean kitchen was finally a pleasant place to make and store food, she wouldn't resort to restaurants and fast food so frequently. She even realized she had room to create an exercise area.

The starting point for change is the vision you hold in your mind for the life you want to live. That is where our focus will be. It's time for a clean start. It's time to reimagine your life.

START BIG — DEFINE YOUR VISION

Every aspect of life is interconnected — how we act, what we own, where we live, what we put into our bodies. You can't deal with the fat on your body if you are trapped in a home that is smothering under the fat of what you own. To deal with your own weight, you need to open up the spaces around you so that your world is lighter. If clutter and disorganization are even a small part of your life, this is where the work starts.

FOOD-CLUTTER PRINCIPLE

Imagine the life you want and hold that idea in your mind as you work through the process.

IMAGINE THE LIFE YOU WANT TO LIVE

Very few things in life are black and white. This is true for both clutter and weight issues. My experience, and that of so many people I've worked with, is that clutter and weight are closely linked. I can't tell you scientifically how one influences the other, but in my experience many, many of the people who struggle with their weight also struggle with balance in other areas of their life — most frequently where another form of buying or consuming is involved. I've received hundreds and hundreds of e-mails from people telling me about the connection they see and experience between clutter and their weight; so many that I don't think it's a coincidence.

So, back to you. Forget about food for a moment and work through this with me — even if it seems silly or unrealistic. We are first going to look at one kind of excess in your life — the clutter in your home.

This is our stepping-off point. Pause for a moment and really think about this question:

What is the life I want to live?

I cannot think of a question that has had more impact on the lives of the people with whom I've worked. Life is never perfect, but we all have unique visions of the life we wish was ours. When clutter fills your home, not only does it block your space, but it also blocks your vision — literally and metaphorically. With every new client I rediscover that at some stage people stop seeing the clutter — even when they can't see over it! They move around it as though it were not there. Asking this question is a way of taking you beyond the clutter, the mess, the lack of organization, to look at your life from a fresh perspective: how you picture your place in the world. "What is the life I want?" It's a deceptively simple question and one that we seldom ask.

From the question "What is the life I want?" flows a range of related questions that you need to seriously ponder. In this imagined life, how do you spend your time? How do you look? How do you feel when you're at home? What does your home look like? The rooms in your home? Your career? How do you feel when you wake up in the morning? What do you eat? How do you spend your time? What is your daily routine? What are you easily able to physically achieve? What do you accomplish in your home? Do you see yourself as high-powered, successful, and organized? What are your relationships like in this imagined life? Do you imagine a rich family life where everyone hangs out together? How do you interact? How do you relax? How do you have fun? What do you do when you come home at night? What do you come home to? Do you hope to one day find a perfect balance of work and home, of stimulation and calm?

What does this ideal life look like? Defining your vision for the life you want is the start of deciding what is of value to you and what you need to let go.

Define your vision for the life you want to live

Words that describe the life I want to live:

- ▪ _____

- ▪ _____

- ▪ _____

- ▪ _____

- ▪ _____

- ▪ _____

Describe what your ideal life would be like:

_____

_____

_____

These are questions that most of us don't get around to asking ourselves. We accept how we are and find it hard to imagine things any other way. Sure, every once in a while something triggers a response in us and we try to change one part of our lives or another. We get up earlier to exercise — for a week at least. We stop eating carbs — until we go out to dinner and can't help but devour the bread rolls. We clear the junk mail from the kitchen table — but leave it on the kitchen counter until we decide what to do with it. Our intentions are good, and the first step is undertaken with enthusiasm, but the follow-through . . . well, we all know about the follow-through.

Change is hard. It is much easier to leave things as they are than it is to take action. This is especially true if you are burdened with a sense of failure at not being able to achieve the goals you set for yourself. Well, this is the day when all that changes! It may take some time and some serious reflection to imagine the life you want to live. The details may be slow in coming to your mind. Don't worry, this is not unusual. Most of us aren't in the habit of really taking the time to contemplate the details of an imagined reality. But having a fully formed image of your ideal life is key to making progress and worth the investment of some quiet time. Give yourself some time so you can really think through what it is you want from this one life that you have.

YOUR IDEAL YOU

Clutter can rob you of the happiness and joy to which you are entitled. The same is true when it comes to an out-of-shape and over-weight body. When you imagine the life you want, don't think about your ideal weight as a number on a scale. Think about achieving a sense of happiness and well-being. Think about how you will feel, how you will spend your time, what you can achieve, and how you can interact with those around you. Your life is so much more than your waist measurement — keep that in mind as you work to develop a fully realized dream of who you can be.

Imagine not just what you *have* but what you *are.* Imagine your body. What does this body of yours look like? How does it feel on the outside and on the inside? How does it function? What can it achieve? What does it do well? How does it relate to others? When you are working on the next activity, think about what happiness is for you. Don't assume that being thin will fix everything. Blame your weight for the problems it truly causes, and take responsibility for fixing those problems. However, be sensible about what you can achieve. You may fantasize about running a marathon, and that's great.

Be my guest. But don't make that a goal for your ideal self unless you really need to run marathons in order to be happy.

ACTIVITY

Imagine your ideal you

How would these parts of my life be different for the ideal me?

Home: _____

Health: _____

Emotions: _____

Relationships: _____

Career: _____

The Gap Between Real and Ideal

Imagining the body you want can be difficult. It's easy to pick out your favorite movie star or model and say, "Jennifer Aniston. I want *her* body," or "That guy in the underwear commercial — that's a six-pack I want." But come on, let's be realistic. You can't compete with fame, fortune, and airbrushing. Instead, think in terms of how your discontent with your body affects how you live in the world. Have you been hiding behind baggy, unflattering clothes? Is that really how you want to live? What do you *want* to wear? And don't tell me you want to model bikinis. We've all been taunted by those stereotypes more than we can stand. Enough already! Instead, focus on being the best you can be. What does that person really look like?

Dear Peter:

I'd wanted all my life to be thin. Growing up with a mother who told me I was fat when I really wasn't, and in a sometimes violent family, led to all kinds of emotional attachments to food. But I became very clear in this new uncluttered home that it was time to feel as good about my body as I now felt about our home. I began adding to my meditations — releasing all unnecessary cells in my body, letting go of whatever I didn't totally NEED in order to survive, live a long life, and manifest my purpose in this lifetime. I've created a vision board of how I want to look — I'm 5'3" and three weeks ago was 203 pounds! I'm now about 192 and for the first time finding it way easier to eat properly, get clear about why food has been instinctively comforting, and get rid of whatever I don't really need. At age fifty-five I probably don't want to be the 135 pounds I once craved. That might leave me with a few too many wrinkles. But I have this quiet confidence and belief that I'm going to declutter and finally reveal the true ME that I've been covering up with food most of my life. The exhilaration of purging/sorting/living light has definitely inspired me to achieve the same euphoria about my body and the way I look.

If you truly want to change, you need to have a clear image of a realistic goal. Pick sensible goals and commit to achieving your vision. Let's talk more about what goals make sense.

How Do You Know Your Ideal Weight?

We have all heard it, said it, or thought it at one time or another: "I need to lose ten pounds," or "I have to fit into these jeans," or "I'll start at the gym on Monday," or "No more bread — ever!" We all have a fixation with losing weight, but have you ever stopped to ask yourself why? What is it that weighing less will give you? What do you expect from "skinny"?

How do you imagine your life would be different at this ideal weight you're seeking?

Your healthy, fit body should help you create the life you imagine for yourself. It should set you on the path toward your goals. Instead of scales or tables or advice from an expert, imagine that life. Now try this. Instead of thinking of a dream weight or a number of pounds to lose, imagine what it is you would be able to do differently at your ideal weight.

Let me help you out a bit. Consider these characteristics of the ideal you: You have relationships that are built on trust and mutual respect; you are a healthy weight that you can maintain; you have established sound and regular eating patterns; your schedule allows you the time to pursue activities that you enjoy; regular exercise is a part of your daily routine; fear does not govern your life; you have a balance between the social, spiritual, psychological, and physical aspects of your life; you accept and love the person you are.

Here are some goals that people who visited my website have shared with me.

SAMPLE GOALS FOR MY IDEAL BODY

With my ideal body I will be able to:

- Walk to the grocery store without losing my breath
- Fit in an airplane seat without a seat belt extender
- Feel pretty/handsome when I wake up
- Walk around the block with my grandchildren
- Look at pictures of myself without getting embarrassed
- Walk up the stairs without becoming winded
- Stop having pain in my knees
- Stop taking blood pressure medicine that is weight related
- Wear a bathing suit without feeling self-conscious
- Tuck my shirt into my pants and wear a pretty belt without my fat tummy hanging out!
- Hike Diamond Head without getting winded
- Spend a ridiculous amount of money on a Burberry outfit (not just the shoes and handbags)
- Stop seeing my closet and mirrors as the enemy

Now that you've read others' goals, let's hear some of your own:

ACTIVITY

Establish goals for your ideal body

With my ideal body I will be able to:

■

_____

■

_____

■

_____

■

_____

Focus on achieving those things that create happiness and well-being in your life. Your goal is not a magic number but a weight that enables you to live your life as you wish.

You are who you are — a gift that should be celebrated. Accepting who you are is a fundamental part of finding happiness. This can be a real challenge in a society that says to be happy you need to be thin, have a lot of money, perfect teeth, and drive the latest car. Stay focused on your image of an ideal you. That image should be defined by *the best you can be.* Look inward and explore what is possible. Reaching your goal will involve change and sacrifice, but you can do it. I have seen countless people achieve their ideal in their homes, their bodies, and their lives, and I know you can, too.

Don't Let Fat Get in the Way

When I help people get rid of sentimental clutter, I remind them that the object is not the memory. In the same way, you are not your fat! Even though you may have identified with being overweight for most of your life, change is possible. Change and the unknown are frightening. For some the very thought of change can be so paralyzing that it stops them from taking any action at all. Fear of change can also be tied up with fear of failure — you've tried so often to lose weight and every time you've failed. Why go through an exercise in futility all over again? Understand that this feeling is not at all unusual or uncommon. We have been led to believe that people can easily change their weight — they do it all the time in infomercials, on reality shows, and in the endless before and after stories in magazines. It must naturally follow, then, that if you cannot be just like them, the problem must be you. Not so.

The *you* that you aspire to be must be nurtured and you must allow your true self to be revealed. This can only be done by establishing and maintaining a place of calm within your life where you are happy with who you are and comfortable with the body you have.

Understand this: If you don't strive to achieve your ideal you, no one else will. So you have failed a few times — welcome to the human race! Now this time, let's make it happen for you.

Make the time

It's easy to have a vision. Now you need to make room for it. Changes take commitment and commitment takes time. I know, I know. You're too busy to be healthy. You have a hectic life. You barely have time to go to the bathroom, much less figure out what changes you need to make to your diet. You eat on the run. You skip meals. You do whatever you can to get by. Heck, even reading this book is taking too long. Enough already.

FOOD-CLUTTER PRINCIPLE

The fat didn't appear overnight and won't disappear overnight.

Sure, you're busy. Here's some breaking news: Everybody's busy. We all have lots of commitments. We all work hard. We all have family and friends and social obligations. Take a look around you. See that fit guy who services your car? He's really busy, too! See that slender businesswoman going into a meeting across the hall? She works later than you do. How do they do it? Lucky genes? Occasionally. But mostly they've learned the time paradox.

There's never enough time,
and there's always more time.

You *can* find the time. It does exist, I promise you.

Time that doesn't serve your goals

Hating your body is time-consuming. How long does it take you to get dressed in the morning? Do you ever change clothes, looking for the perfect outfit that is flattering and flab-hiding, eventually settling on black because, as we all know, black is slimming? Do you stand in front of the mirror with your belly sucked in, convincing yourself that you can go the whole evening without exhaling? Have you given up on your body, instead spending hours in front of the mirror perfecting your hair and your face, or focusing

96

on your manicure and pedicure? When you go shopping, is it hard for you to find the right clothes, clothes that hide problems but still suit your personal style? Do you go into store after store, never quite finding what you're looking for? It's ironic, isn't it, that being unsatisfied with your body means you spend so much time focusing on it?

Look at your daily schedule. If you have a job, part of your work time is fixed; you have to sleep every night; you have set commitments. The rest of your time is up for grabs. Are you spending your time in ways that serve the life you want to live? You say you don't have time to cook. What exactly are you doing while you wait for the takeout to arrive or the frozen food to thaw? Watching TV? Say hello to your cooking time. My client Brooke is a single working woman. She spends at least fifteen hours a week watching TV, mostly, as she calls them, "cheesy reality shows." When I asked her what purpose it served, she said that it gave her a feeling of pleasure and relaxation like nothing else. She loves TV and most of us, including me, agree that it's a pretty great invention. Brooke and I talked about how important TV was to her and weighed it against how much she hated being fat. She said, "I'd throw away my TV tonight if it meant I'd wake up skinny." We both knew that wasn't going to happen, but Brooke realized that she was willing to compromise on her TV watching. She vowed to stop eating frozen dinners and brought a TV into her kitchen to watch while she made meals from scratch. Several weeks later she called me and said, "It's working! I've lost four pounds. And next week I have my first date in three years. I'm going to miss *American Idol,* but who cares?"

TV FACTS

Nearly a quarter of adults say they have no physical activity at all in their leisure time and the average teenager spends close to six hours a day in front of a screen of some sort — close to an hour each online and playing video games and another four hours watching TV. The average child spends twenty-eight hours a week in front of the TV and the average adult about thirty-one hours a week doing the same. This amounts to more than two months of continuous TV viewing every year.

It's amazing how a little TV here and there adds up. If these numbers seem crazy to you, do your own calculations:

ACTIVITY

Calculate how much time a year you spend in front of the TV

The number of hours I usually watch TV on a weekday = ☐

x 5

Total number of TV hours on weekdays = ___

The number of hours I usually watch TV on a Saturday: + ☐

The number of hours I usually watch TV on a Sunday: + ☐

Total number of hours a week = ___

x 52

Total number of hours a year: ___

Circle the number of hours you watch TV a year in the lefthand column of the table below. How many weeks of continuous TV viewing is this a year? How many months? Are you off the scale?

TELEVISION WATCHING SCALE		
HOURS	WEEKS	MONTHS
168	1	
336	2	
504	3	
672	4	1
840	5	
1008	6	
1176	7	
1344	8	2
1512	9	
1680	10	
1848	11	
2016	12	3

Give up TV

You heard me. I said: Give up TV. Before you throw this book out the window, just try it for a month. Tape your favorite show, if you must. If time is at a premium, isn't it worth it to know what it would feel like to change your TV habits? TV is the biggest rut that we all fall into. What would life be like without it? You owe it to yourself to find out. Think of your no-TV time as a gift to yourself. Use the time to plan activities you never have enough time to do: filing papers, reading a book, calling an old friend, going to the gym, hosting a dinner party. Or don't plan anything. See where the time leads you. (But, whatever you do, don't let your free time lead you to the refrigerator.)

Since you'll have so much extra time, jot down a log showing things you accomplish during your former TV hours. Take note of how it makes you feel to have so much free time. See if it affects how often you prepare dinner, how much you enjoy it, and how much you eat. At the end of the month you'll have a rare opportunity —

the opportunity to make an active choice about how much TV you want in your life instead of passively letting it consume your evenings.

Invest time on the ideal you

Look for ways to make your time more efficient. Do you spend a good chunk of your day taking care of your children? How can you make that time active? If you're chauffeuring them to soccer practice, can you take a brisk walk or jog around the field while you wait to take them home? (Or around the block if you don't want to embarrass them.) Are you spending time shopping for food? Make good choices. Are you spending time shopping for clothes and material goods? Give it up. You have enough. Too much. And you know it.

Stop multitasking

Ever had a friend take a cell phone call during dinner or done so yourself? Ever sat next to a date in a movie theater while one or both of you checked your PDAs? Ever found yourself in a business meeting where everyone was simultaneously on their PDAs while "listening" to a presenter? Ever checked e-mail while on the phone? Ever been on the phone while you walked the dog? Ever watched TV while you cooked? Ever read a magazine while you ate? Fixed your hair or makeup while driving? Paid bills while you tried to read to your child? Multitasking has become a way of life. At first it sounds like a compliment: "He's a multitasker. He can do three things at once." You should hire the guy, right? Wrong. When you're multitasking your concentration is split and something always loses out. Think about what happens to your ability to drive when you're talking on the phone. Other activities don't have the high-risk, split-second danger of driving, but the damage, while less dramatic, can still be as significant.

What's the rush? What are you accomplishing by doing everything half-assed? Live your life in the present. Be where you are. Be mindful. Be *respectful*. If you are watching TV and eating, which activity do you think wins more of your attention? And what happens if you're not eating mindfully? I'll tell you. You just keep going, past when you're full, past enjoyment — that is, if you ever even bothered to notice the taste of your food. Just try it.

Stop multitasking for a week

Three ways I multitask	Which task is more important?	What I have to do to make the change?
1.		
2.		
3.		

Enjoy the time that good choices create

My friend Leela spends hours at the gym every morning. One day I asked her what her goal was — she worked so hard. Was she trying to lose weight, or be stronger, or what? She said, "Are you kidding? I go for the same reason every morning: to burn off the guilt of last night's dessert." If you've ever watched those calorie counters on machines at the gym you know that it takes hours and hours to burn off just a few calories. Eating whatever you want and then going to the gym doesn't work, no matter how hard you work out. You'll never get ahead. Once I overheard some personal trainer telling his client that fitness is 90 percent what you eat and 10 percent exercise. I don't care if it's scientifically true, but I buy it. You're wasting time if you're trying to burn guilt calories. How does guilt fit into the life you want to live? Guilt is a waste of time. Take control of your life and you won't have guilt.

When you truly prioritize your time you'll be surprised at what happens. Stop spending time on things that aren't important to you and time emerges for the things that are. Build on the life you want. If you're like many people and spend two months a year watching TV, take steps now to reclaim that time. If you spend less time shopping for clothes and household items that you don't need and more time getting organized and creating your best life, you'll start to find that the bills are paid, there's a healthy dinner on the table, and you're excited to go out on Friday night and show off on the dance floor.

PRACTICE MINDFUL EATING

When you create time, when you stop multi-tasking, when you isolate your experiences, you are finally free to find joy in all aspects of your day. Know what you are doing and why you are doing it. Know where you are. Be who you are. When you bring these principles to meals, to where, when, how, why, and with whom you eat, you will change your whole relationship with food.

We've talked about the life you want to live. We've talked about setting priorities and investing your time in that life. That's all fine and good, you say, but what do I do? Where do I begin? How does it really work? Can I really take the vision I have for the life I want and make that real? The answer is absolutely, positively yes, you can!

As I have said earlier, there are not a lot of secrets and certainly no magic to the work I do with my clients. About 90 percent of what I say and do with clients is good old-fashioned common sense. You have common sense, too. I believe you instinctively know what needs to be done. Maybe, just maybe, it's time to listen to that inner voice you've been ignoring. It's time to apply some of your own good old-fashioned common sense to a problem that has gotten way out of control.

Be honest with yourself. Admit what you know in your heart — it has taken years for you to get to where you are and change cannot happen overnight. Anyone who tells you so is offering false hope, guaranteeing something they simple cannot deliver, and ensuring certain failure. That said, what *can* change overnight is that you can come to understand what actions have gotten you where you are and why you behave the way you do. You can learn to take the first steps to choosing another healthier way for yourself, your children, and your whole family.

Now that you have the vision for the life you want, it's time to look at your emotions, your home, your kitchen, your food, and your meals, and the place that food has in your life. Clutter in any of these areas — geography, habits, routines, or lifestyle choices — affects your mood, your outlook, and your weight. Getting rid of that clutter is the route to happiness.

You are well on your way. The solution is in your hands.

CHECKLIST FOR CHAPTER TWO

- ❏ Define your vision of the life you want to live.
- ❏ Imagine your ideal you.
- ❏ Establish goals for your ideal body.
- ❏ Estimate your TV-watching time per year.
- ❏ Stop watching TV for a month.
- ❏ Stop multitasking for a week.

Three:
The Emotions
You Confront

MIND OVER MOOD

Food has meaning. It keeps us alive. It tastes good. Eating is part of your practical life and your relationships. But in the same way that clutter takes over your life and has power over you, food takes on many different meanings. Your relationship with food is as complex as you are. Why? Because for many of us food has become symbolic. It's there when we're happy. It's there when we're sad. And over the years we connect it to those emotions and all the emotions in between. Consequently, we eat food — usually unhealthy food — for many reasons beyond hunger.

When fears and doubts crop up, it makes perfect sense to turn to food, which you and your body identify in the most primal way as a means of sustenance. Not only do we eat when we're hungry, but also we eat whenever we feel a specific emotion, be it loneliness, happiness or celebration, boredom, fear, anger, need for comfort, for reward, and on and on. Over time, we develop habits. We eat when confronted with particular emotions. These food triggers are personal clutter that most of us have. What we're eating no longer has anything to do with food as pleasure or sustenance. Instead, it's the answer to the wrong kind of hunger: an attempt to fill a void that can never be filled.

Dear Peter:

I have my vision for my house. Maybe I need a vision for my body. I will be fifty next year. I want to have my body and house in order by then. I hope it doesn't take that long. I believe my weight and clutter problems are only outward manifestations of my inner clutter. I have been dealing with so many losses in my life and I really believe the clutter is a way of filling my emptiness.

I had a weird experience the other day that made me think that way. I actually cleaned off the two dressers in my bedroom. When I did, the room felt empty to me, even though I had a nice flower arrangement on both dressers.

Maybe you already know your emotional triggers, but sometimes they can be tough to pin down. Let's look at your daily life to identify some of the most common emotional triggers that can cause you to lose control and stop making choices. Certain places, interactions, or moments of the day can help you figure out where these triggers are hiding.

Where do you eat?

Is a certain place or places one of your triggers for unhealthy eating? Where you eat is a major clue to what emotions lead you to food.

- Do you eat in secret at home? This could mean you're lonely or depressed. It could mean your home stresses you out.
- Do you eat on the run or in fast-food restaurants? Maybe for you food is tied to the anxiety of an overbooked schedule and a life that feels out of control. Eating quickly feels like your only option.
- Do you eat perfectly well all day . . . until you pass the same convenience store on your way home from work and find yourself unable to resist buying a

candy bar just because it's there? Is that candy bar a reward? A treat you're giving yourself because you don't feel happy? Is it a way you can feel in control because nobody can tell you not to buy that candy?

Don't pull the trigger

Start by exploring what makes you weak in your trigger moment. Are you eating because the food is free and available? Do you convince yourself that eating a certain way means it doesn't "count"? Are you eating because you're someplace that feels special, so you "deserve to splurge"? When a place is your trigger, it is often about instant gratification. You know you could hold out for healthy food, but that hamburger is right here, right now. It's sitting in front of you. You know it will be satisfying. We search for instant gratification to fill a hole. What is the hole? What is missing from your life that makes you so determined to prove to yourself that what you want can be yours?

To break the place trigger, you have to put a new routine in place. The new routine can be food-related — carry a healthy snack and eat it whenever you enter the trigger place. Or it can be activity-related — call a certain friend to stop you from responding to the trigger. In the same way that you need to be mindful of what you put into your body, you need to eat in places that are conducive to good health and healthy choices. Where can you eat and be aware of what you're putting into your body? That's right. At a table, with food that you prepare, fully engaged with those around you.

When do you eat?

Is the time of day a clue to your emotional trigger?

- Do you have a consistent, reliable schedule, or is every week full of unexpected changes in plans? Do you have fixed mealtimes? Or do you wait until you're starving and then grab the first snack you see? A life in flux makes us seek the stability of comfort foods.

- Do you snack in mid-afternoon? A pick-me-up is literally that — a desperate attempt to find energy when you have none left. Why are you so depleted? What is running you ragged? Unless you have a physically strenuous job, you shouldn't be so exhausted by mid-afternoon that without a candy bar you won't survive. Are there problems at work that wear you down?

- Do you eat healthy food all day and then come home to indulge? This is a sign of "reward" food.

Don't pull the trigger

You need to stop relying on food to get you through life's harder moments or to reward you for surviving them. You need to deal with the root of the problem. Why is your life so exhausting or challenging? What can you do to bring order and a sane pace to your day.

More immediate, the practical solution is organization. Don't be the person who, at the end of her life, has traded her health, good looks, and (let's take it all the way) self-esteem for some meetings that ran late. So many people I work with can organize their professional lives incredibly well but fall to pieces when it comes to their personal needs or responsibilities. You need to organize your meals, even those you eat away from home or when alone. Don't eat on the run. Ever. You know in advance that you're going to be out, so bring lunch with you. Build a nutritious, energizing snack into your mid-afternoons. If you're going to eat out, make sure there's a healthy option. Even fast-food restaurants are making efforts to provide low-calorie, healthier meals, so you do have options.

It's time to invent new routines. Routines

are important. Create new patterns and habits, ones that serve your goals. The first of these should be to establish mealtimes. If your schedule changes every day, affix the meals to your schedule as best you can ("I always eat breakfast half an hour after I wake up." "I always eat dinner immediately after I get home from work"). By doing this, you'll identify conflicts in your schedule. For example, you're always starving when you get home from work, but of course dinner isn't ready yet, so you snack as you prepare something. Wrong. If you won't have time to prepare dinner when you come home from work, prepare it in advance. Same thing goes if you can't eat until your kids go to school or go down for naps. Know the times of day you need to eat. Plan to have healthy foods that fuel your ideal life. Keep that life in mind. Would you rather be mildly to totally unhappy about your body for life or be a healthy weight for life? Every day that you live is made up of choices like these. You are not helpless.

How much and how fast do you eat?

In this age of supersizing, there are whole books about portion size. Restaurants serve us twice what we need and it's hard to know when to stop. If you eat healthy foods but are still overweight, you need to explore what makes you overeat. Do you crave a sensation of excess — you want to feel like you can have as much as you want. You want more, more, more and once you start, you just can't stop. Why are you eating on autopilot? Where is your head when you raise the fork to your mouth? Is something distracting you? Or is eating an escape, and you want that feeling to last as long as possible?

Don't pull the trigger

Years ago my very good friend Greg got into the habit of asking waiters at restaurants to serve him only half of his main course and to put the other half into a take-out container. He never wastes any food, controls the amount he eats, and always has a second meal for the following day. As you probably know by now, I'm not a big fan of scales or measures. The best way to judge an appropriate portion size is to put together a nice, modest-looking plate and not to eat more than that. Don't ever eat from a big bag of chips or a carton of ice cream, promising yourself that you're only going to have a little. Serve it out, and no second helpings.

When it comes to how fast you eat, don't bother timing yourself. Just slow down. Try to taste each bite. Savor your food. Give yourself a good twenty minutes before you go back for seconds. It takes time for your body to realize it's full.

Dear Peter:
   I began to collect things at about the time my oldest children began leaving home. I think I was trying to replace something missing from my life. Same with food; I eat not because I am necessarily hungry, but because I am trying to fill a void. I know that I need to get my life (and my home) back on track. I have always WANTED to be organized, even as a child, but find reasons why I "can't" be (not enough time, space, money, know-how). I know I am rationalizing when I do this and I want to stop.

HOW YOU FEEL BEFORE, DURING, AND AFTER YOU EAT

Many different emotions lead to overeating: the need for comfort after a long, tiring day; a sense of loneliness or emptiness that feels like it could be filled with food; a feeling that you deserve a reward for success or hard work; exhaustion; anger; hopelessness; despair . . . the list is endless. All of these emotions are real and they are important and they deserve your attention. Food is one way of giving them attention, and it helps — temporarily — because you get an infusion of energy that can lift you out of a mood. But food never gets to the heart of the problem. If you don't get to the heart of the problem, it doesn't go away. And if it doesn't go away, you find yourself using food to self-medicate over and over again. So don't ignore your emotions, face them straight on and work through them.

Activity: A New Kind of Food Journal

As we explore triggers further, I'll help you identify yours and I'll do my best to help you establish new patterns to detach those emotions from the act of eating. Sometimes triggers aren't easy to pin down, and the best way to identify a trigger as subtle as an emotion is to make a note after you've eaten something you regret. I want you to try keeping a food diary. Wait! I know almost every nutritionist and every diet book out there asks people to keep a food diary. Why? What's the point? Either you're cheating — in which case who wants to admit it? Or you're eating perfectly — in which case, why do you need to document it? But I want you to keep a journal not to track your food intake but to track where you go wrong. When you do make unhealthy choices, note where you ate, how much you ate, why you ate, and how you felt when you were eating. It's a hard thing to do, because you're essentially confessing to yourself. But that honest information is the best way to identify the emotion — or emotions — that triggered your slip.

Once you identify the emotions, you can start taking the necessary steps to make a change. Some of these emotions are powerful and to address them may require hard work. It's your choice.

I don't need you to write down every thing that you eat all day long. I want you to use your journal to confront your food triggers head-on and you won't be able to unless you document honestly every time you eat unwisely and why you did it. I'll tell you why. We human beings are simple creatures. Some of the time we are rational, in-control creatures. But much of the time we have conflicting desires. We want to eat well, but we want to eat huge slabs of pizza. So what do we do? We find ways to justify our irrational decisions. The most popular lie we tell ourselves is "I'll start tomorrow." Runners-up are: "I only had a little"; "I was good all day so I deserve dessert"; and "I worked out today so I can eat whatever I want." Those excuses, and any others you can think of, are why a food and activity journal can be a lifesaver. I want you to learn to be a mindful eater, but if your brain and your stomach seem to have conflicting interests, there's no better way to get them to communicate with each other than to write it down in black and white. No more lies.

Keep track of those moments when you turn to food for reasons other than satisfying your hunger at mealtimes. So you ate an entire pint of Ben & Jerry's? Instead of feeling guilty and giving up, I want you to tell the story of the moment leading up to that decision. Where were you? What time was it? What were you feeling? How was your day? Was the food satisfying? Did it make you feel good? How did you feel half an hour later? Energized or bloated? Is that a feeling you want to have again? What can your body tell you about your weight? Write it down. Then forgive yourself and start again. If that was your only lapse, congratulations! But if you find yourself returning to your old habits, start looking at the pattern that is forming in your food diary. What is behind the moment of decision? Is it an emotion? Is it a habit at a certain time of day? Are you making a bad choice because you didn't have a plan? Is it a perfect storm of events — you're tired, home late from work, and angry at your boss for keeping you overtime? Or maybe your trigger is an ongoing struggle.

Use your journal to be honest and to rethink your choices. Use it to teach yourself to be mindful. And don't quit your journal even if you eat an entire gallon of ice cream. Keep going, and we'll get to the root of the ice-cream problem.

FOOD-CLUTTER PRINCIPLE
Live in the present, not the past or the future. If you're eating for emotional reasons, figure out why. Anger? Despair? Comfort? Fear?

ACTIVITY	
Identify the triggers that lead to overeating	
TRIGGERS THAT LEAD ME TO OVEREAT	
Internal triggers	External triggers

Confront the trigger

Once you know your trigger, now what can you do? You need to confront it head-on. But I want you to approach it in two different ways. The first is to deal with the emotion itself. Where is the feeling of anger or loneliness or emptiness coming from? How can you change that? Do you need to make changes in your life? The emotional triggers that lead to overeating are often old wounds that run deep. In many ways these triggers are not so different from the clutter that fills our homes. They come into our lives and fill our spaces. Over time, we stop being able to see them clearly or to get rid of them easily. In the same way that strong memories or deep fears are tied to physical clutter, it's not unusual for this emotional clutter to be closely tied to your food habits. You're not going to solve them instantaneously by reading a paragraph in a book. There is work to be done, whether by yourself, with your partner and/or friends, or with a professional. An imbalanced relationship with food doesn't have a place in your best life. At the very least, overeating is a hurdle to achieving the life you want. At its worst it's life threatening. You can't invest time in any better work than this. It's an investment toward the life you want for yourself.

> Dear Peter:
> On the outside I'm well-groomed, dress nicely, and I'm a nice, fun person. I think where I struggle is that I'm fearful of taking that next step, wondering what it would be like to be fifty pounds lighter and to have my home and life in order.

The second approach, which happens at the same time, can have an immediate effect. It's simple, and it's what I've been describing all along. Use new routines to stop pulling the trigger. Plan for the outcome you want. Focus and work on the behaviors that suit you best. You can throw those emotional triggers for a loop by putting new, healthy habits in their way. It's much easier to resist that pint of ice cream when you've already filled up on healthy food and you have the energy that comes from regular, balanced meals

BUILD NEW HABITS

Have a plan

Routines help reinforce the habits you want. Those habits help create the body you're after. Knowing where your next meal is coming from and what it's going to be is critical to weight loss. We eat bad food when we let ourselves get too hungry to take the time to prepare healthy food. If your desk is organized, you'll work more efficiently. If your time is scheduled, you won't be late. If you check a map, you won't get lost (in theory anyway). If you buy your plane tickets in advance, you'll (usually) save money. You know the drill. If you plan your meals, you'll fill your hungry self with healthy options. Haven't you ever noticed that when you prepare a real meal for yourself, a meal that looks colorful on the plate and leaves you feeling satisfied, you feel better about yourself? When you honor and respect your body, you feel proud and more attractive. You've made a commitment to a healthy, happy life. In Chapter 6 you'll learn how to support this healthy life with a healthy menu that you create and implement.

Variation and moderation

Lots of people quit diets because they get "bored." Sure, you're going to get bored if you make the same salad for lunch every day for a month. The hardest thing to do when you're cooking for yourself is to branch out. Branching out means seeking variety by tracking down new recipes. It means buying unfamiliar ingredients and trying new things. It means taking a little longer to prepare your food because you're not used to making it. But that's what planning is all about. Mix in new meals with staples. I'm going to want you to make a shopping list anyway, so it's not that much extra work. Try new cuisines. Buy vegetables you've passed up for years in the grocery store. (If you have no idea whether an item should be boiled or roasted, ask someone at the store for guidance on preparation.) Interesting food is more satisfying. Variety is the spice of life — and more nutritious, too. Variety is tied to moderation. An entire bag of Pirate's Booty is not a meal. A large order of french fries is not a meal. But a roasted chicken breast with a vegetable and a few french fries *is* a meal. It's easy to overeat your favorite foods, but when you balance them with more nutritious and satisfying foods, you're less likely to binge.

Pick new behaviors to substitute for your emotional triggers. Mix and match from the examples below or make up your own.

Find healthy substitutions

INSTEAD OF:	I WILL:
Snacking when I'm bored . . .	Walk for fifteen minutes.
Rewarding myself after a hard day with a pint of ice cream . . .	Pick a small, manageable area of my house (a drawer, a bookshelf) and fill a bag of stuff for charity.
Eating to relieve stress . . .	Take a bath.
Having a three-hour dinner in front of the TV . . .	Make plans to dine with a friend, or even have a phone date while I eat an amount I decide in advance.
Ignoring my body until tomorrow because those salty treats are here today . . .	Throw away the chips and celebrate by steaming some vegetables.

Find healthy substitutions

INSTEAD OF:	I WILL:
Sneaking down to the kitchen for a midnight snack . . .	Strip down and stand in front of a full-length mirror, reminding myself to treat my body with honor and respect until the urge passes.

For some people it's easier to substitute foods instead of behaviors. Try writing down your worst indulgences and then pick healthy, filling foods or a fun activity as a new and better substitute.

ACTIVITY	
INSTEAD OF EATING:	I WILL EAT:
French fries	A side salad
Ice cream	Plain yogurt with honey

Adopt a secret role model

Look around. No matter who you are and what life you live, if you can look around your workplace, your house of worship, or your community, you will find someone else in your exact situation who is making healthier choices than you are. It could be someone you love and respect, who seems to have a balanced, healthy relationship with food. Of course, maybe it's that annoying waif who never takes more than a bite of the dessert you're "sharing." Maybe it's the marathoner next door who always seems to be eating an apple. I'm certainly not advising you to turn into someone who annoys you or to start running marathons, but I want you to notice the people around you who have found a way to make their relationship with food work. It shows, doesn't it? If they can do it, so can you. That close friend of yours who never has bread before dinner? She's on to something. What else do you notice about the way she eats? How is it different from what you do? Does she always have a salad first? Does she ask for dressing on the side? Does she leave food on her plate? How often does she seem to exercise? What is her attitude at dinner? Is she enjoying her meal? Does she eat slower or more quickly than you? Does she drink more or less? Have dessert sometimes or never? One bite or a whole piece of pie? Don't become a creepy stalker, but remember that all of our eating habits came from somewhere. We developed them as a child, in relationships, in loneliness, and out of hunger. Now is the time to reinvent your relationship with food. Look for models you respect and learn from their behavior. Imitate them enough and eventually it won't feel forced. You won't feel like a copycat faker because you'll have new habits, a new attitude, and, eventually, a new body to match. Before you know it, you'll have someone imitating you!

Adopt a Secret Food Role Model

Role Model No. 1:	What I admire about this person:	What I want to imitate:
Role Model No. 2:	What I admire about this person:	What I want to imitate:

CHECKLIST FOR CHAPTER THREE

- ❏ Identify triggers that lead to overeating.
- ❏ Try a new kind of food journal.
- ❏ Find healthy substitutions.
- ❏ Adopt a secret food role model.

FOUR:
THE HOME WHERE
YOU LIVE

TIME TO COME CLEAN

In my book *It's All Too Much,* I explain how your home is a reflection of you. The space where you live should reflect the life you want to live. Does it? That book breaks down the decisions room-by-room to help readers organize and declutter their homes. When it comes to weight loss, I believe the work begins by making your home an environment where you can relax and enjoy the space you have. I've heard this over and over again from clients and readers who write in to share their experiences. Finding your way out of the clutter helps you take control of your life.

Dear Peter:

I've noticed that when clutter creeps in, it creates a low level of stress. It's almost like the hum of street noise: above my sensory threshold, but below my conscious awareness. I'll attend to all of life's loud noises, like work deadlines and car troubles, but not notice the constant background hiss of all the extra stuff. And since I definitely misuse food — that is, I eat not just for sustenance or nourishment, but as a way to unwind, tune out, get a pleasant little buzz at the end of the day — I find myself eating more just to help block that hiss. Once I start overeating, it kicks off a cycle of guilt that only adds even more stress.

If I actually listened to that hiss, by the way, it would be saying, "You are not quite in control."

But when I can break that cycle and clear my space, the noise goes away. I feel powerful and effective and in control of my life. I no longer want to self-medicate, I want to celebrate! The allure of food never quite vanishes, but I view myself as stronger than the compulsion. Plus, I want my physical self to match my improved psyche and surroundings, not weighed down by extra pounds or heavy meals.

It's All Too Much walked you through the challenges and opportunities that each room presents, so I'm not going to repeat myself here. But I just don't believe you can take control of what and how you eat before you make the place where you begin and end the day a happy, comfortable refuge. Only there will you have the energy, power, and self-confidence to make changes.

FOOD-CLUTTER PRINCIPLE
Organizing where, how, and what you eat is the first step toward achieving your ideal body.

IT'S MORE THAN JUST A HOME — IT'S *YOUR* HOME

Take a look around your house or apartment. This is your home. How does it make you feel? Is it a place you like to come home to? Does it give you a sense of calm and peace? Does it make you feel as if no matter what's going on in the outside world you still have this — a place where you are safe and in control?

Dear Peter:

My family has not been invited to step foot into my house in over a year. I won't allow my kids to have company over because I don't want anyone to see my house. My husband complains about how messy the kids are — well, what can he expect when we're so snowed under with garbage ourselves. After having read your book I truly believe that my depression and weight gain are a direct result of my house. I don't even feel I can call it a home when I hate opening the door.

Your home is the center of your life. It's a reflection of who you are and how you choose to live your life. A chaotic home is a sign of troubles. Your home should help you feel centered and focused, motivated and calm. If it doesn't, there's something wrong. Because if you're not taking control of your home — a place where you have 100 percent control — then how are you supposed to manage the other aspects of your life where you don't have as much control?

Dear Peter:

First of all, I never was the kind of person who had clutter piled high on the dining room table and couldn't walk into my room, but I will say that I think EVERYONE has clutter in their home. A lot of us just have come up with ways of hiding it, by stashing it into closets, drawers, and storage rooms. This creates a daily chaos that robs us of precious time, without us even realizing it!

Your book completely changed my life. When I began with the question of what I really wanted for my space, I quickly said, "I want to be able to clean each room in five minutes!" With three little ones, I didn't have any more TIME to spare than that, and to clean up usually took me hours upon hours!

I went on a cleaning rampage. In this tiny apartment I was able to gather together about sixty-five giant trash bags of giveaway items, and we took several trailerloads of stuff to the dump. To tackle my home I just slowly went drawer by drawer, corner by corner, cabinet by cabinet, until my house had been completely purged and organized. Now that I am done, I cannot get over how wonderful my house looks.

Now I have more time to spend with my husband and three darling children because we only take five minutes to clean a room, and they can do most of their toys and room by themselves! Thank you for your wonderful book and making our home such a wonderful place to live and enjoy life in!

A FAT TOUR OF YOUR HOME

Are you ready to take on your weight? Really ready? I want to know that you're committed to living the life you want. Are you? Not if your house is a junk pile. Do you have the home you deserve: a bedroom that is a sanctuary; a living room where you can gather friends and/or family without feeling embarrassed; a closet that contains only clothes that flatter you and make you feel comfortable; an office where you take control of your business and finances and which makes you feel confident about your path?

If you're cheating yourself out of a happy

home, then you're sabotaging your own life. You aren't making choices that serve your goals. So why in the world would you expect yourself to stay true to a plan to clean up your food habits? If you don't respect yourself enough to create a happy space to live, then how can you treat your body with the honor and respect it deserves?

Let's take a look around. Instead of going through every room as I did in *It's All Too Much,* I'm just going to peek at the areas of your house that fill with weight-related clutter. If you've got problems that extend to every nook and cranny of your house, then you should start with *It's All Too Much.*

Front door

Let's start at the beginning. How do you feel when you walk into your home? Is it a place where you're relaxed and happy, a respite from whatever else might be going on in the world? Is it a place where you like to invite friends? Or do you feel overwhelmed — too much stuff and too many projects in various stages of completion. Are there whole rooms or closets you avoid? If you can't get through the front door without feelings of anxiety, well . . . there's no get-out-of-jail-free card. You need to start with your house (and — I have to say it again — you might want to consider picking up *It's All Too Much*).

Bedroom

Your bedroom is the most important room of your house. It sets the tone for your home and drives the energy that fills your space. It should be the place where your relationship thrives. It should be a peaceful retreat. Is there space for you to relax and decompress? Or is it so cluttered with your kids' videos, old magazines, and dirty laundry that it makes you want to head down to the kitchen for a decompression snack?

What about the clothes in your closet? Do they fit the body you have? Do you have sets of "wish" clothes for different weights — some skinny clothes that you hope will fit you again one day although you do nothing to get there? And some baggy clothes for when you're even fatter than you are now? Either way, you're not living the life you have. If you want to lose weight, you have to face the reality of your body. Respect it for what it is today by dressing it in clothes that fit. Eat well for today, so you feel energetic and strong. Don't waste time dreaming, regretting, or shopping. Get your body to a healthy place, and let the clothes follow. Donate the clothes that don't fit you to a charity. They're not helping matters.

Bathroom

What does your bathroom tell you about your relationship with your body? Is there a scale where you weigh yourself every morning, hoping some miracle has made the numbers change even though you're eating the same junk as always? Don't let the pound-here, pound-there fluctuations of daily life delude you. If you want to see changes, you have to make changes. Does your bathroom (or bedroom) have a full-length mirror where you can bravely and honestly assess your naked body? A mirror or a camera is a great way to make yourself face facts. That's you. The way you look is partly genetic and partly a result of how you care for yourself. You can't control genetics, but you can take great care of yourself.

What kind of products lurk on your bathroom shelves and in your medicine cabinet? Have you tried every miracle cellulite cream to hit the market? Do you have one of those knobby scrubbers that supposedly breaks down the fat so you can look thinner without doing anything more than rubbing your thighs in the shower? Is that a loving, respectful way to treat your body? Here's a hint: If it's easy, it doesn't work. Get rid of your easy fixes. It's time to change.

Dear Peter:

I kept buying weight-loss books and videos and gadgets, thinking they would help me lose weight. However, I realized long ago that in the back of my mind, I was buying them thinking that somehow, magically, the purchase would make me thin (without really using the product). Yes, I know it doesn't really work that way, but that's the feeling you get when you have the item in your hands. You think, I'm holding the key in my hands . . . this is finally going to unlock the prison I'm in. I find myself doing that with other things, too. I buy things to make me happy. But they really don't make me happy at all. I was happier NOT having "things." I was happier when I only had a few things to cherish. I see a direct correlation between weight loss and clutter. The more clutter I have, the more weight I gain. It makes perfect sense.

All of the weight-loss products have added to the clutter, too. I think that is where part of the link is — the weight-loss items are creating clutter. The clutter is causing me to be depressed. The depression is causing me to eat. Being overweight is causing me to search for a solution. Searching for the solution is causing me to buy more weight-loss products. And the weight-loss products are still creating more clutter.

Bookshelves

I want you to make a stack of all the diet books and other self-help books on your shelves. How much did they cost? How much do they weigh? How much room do they take up? Get real. Those diets failed you. So why do you still have the books? Because you think that you're the one who failed. Maybe you are. Congratulations, now let's move on. Get rid of the dead weight of fad books that promise miracles. Stop holding on to that extra weight: You don't waste valuable time and space on failures anymore. You make changes.

Exercise paraphernalia

What else did you spend money on, hoping it would make you lose weight? Do you have exercise machines covered in dust? How about workout DVDs? Weights that you never lift? None of these things make you lose weight just by existing. You have to do something. In all my years of decluttering homes, I have never seen a piece of exercise equipment that was used with any regularity. Never! Change can only follow choice. Make a choice now. If you aren't going to use that standing bicycle or ab-crunch machine today, it's gotta go.

Garage

You can't live the life you want if you're focused on the past or on the future. Our garages are full of relics of a past life: thin clothes, photos of our youth, wedding dresses, college football helmets. They are also full of the clutter of an unlived life: sports equipment that doesn't get used, photos where you look too fat so you refuse to put them in albums. Fantasies of a life you haven't lived because you're too busy shopping, watching TV, gaining weight, and otherwise avoiding reality.

Your house is a big project. I can't walk you through it here. But I want you to see how hard it is to change when you don't have the space to do so. I want you to realize how important it is to start your work in a physical space that is under your control. If you can't control what goes into the space around you, you'll never take control of what goes inside your body.

FIVE:
THE KITCHEN YOU CREATE

NOBODY MAKES GOOD CHOICES IN A MESSY KITCHEN

If you walked into a new restaurant and saw a messy, disorganized kitchen and dining area, you'd turn around and walk out the door. You wouldn't eat dinner in a place like that. So why would you do it at home? Let's take a closer look at the parts of your home where you store, prepare, and eat your meals. We want them to make sense. These are the areas of your home that should nourish you and your family. We want them to cater to the life you want.

Dear Peter:

My "stuff" has taken over everything. I purchase tons of food, too. I cook and eat. I think eating makes me happy, but the end result is that I am overweight and my kitchen is usually a mess and the pantry is overflowing so much that you can't walk in front of it. You have to step on food to get to more food. I don't even know what I have in the pantry any longer. So . . . I go purchase more food. I've tried to declutter. I've tried to decrease the activities and I always return to my old ways. I am afraid I have hurt my marriage beyond repair.

Clutter is an obstacle. It impedes your ability to find things, use things, appreciate things, and to leverage the space and materials you have to build a fruitful, rewarding life. People don't cook anymore; that's why 60 percent of us are overweight — because in a restaurant or fast-food place you are served humongous portions of food that are infused with more fat than you could possibly store, much less use for cooking in your kitchen. Have you ever seen a fresh batch of french fries rise up from a vat of boiling oil? Yeah, and have you ever seen that much oil in anybody's home kitchen? I didn't think so.

I have seen that for most people the more they prepare food and cook it at home, the more weight they'll lose. But it's no fun to cook in a messy, disorganized kitchen where you can't find what you need or take pleasure in the process. I want you to cook. I want you to plan for it. I want you to do it mindfully. Let's make your kitchen a place where that can happen.

WHAT DO YOU WANT FROM YOUR KITCHEN?

Every room in your house should have a clear purpose. Some are easy to define. A bathroom is where you use the toilet, clean your body, and perhaps do your hair and makeup. A guest room is where visitors stay. An office is where you handle personal and business affairs. But our lives and our houses have more complicated purposes. The master bedroom is for sleeping. And it's more than that. It's where a couple has private, romantic time together. It's where they establish and maintain the core of their relationship. If a desk enters the master bedroom, everything changes. If children's toys and clothes infiltrate, it tells you something about the fraying of your center. The master bedroom drives the home. It is the heart of the house. It represents stability and love.

If the master bedroom is not in shape, the rest of the household can easily lose direction. Similarly, the kitchen nourishes the home. The kitchen is where it all happens. It's the place where you and your household look for all kinds of sustenance. Kitchens tend to be warm (even though hearths are a thing of the past) and welcoming. Most people find that no matter how much effort they put into decorating the "public" rooms of the house — the living room and dining room — if people come over, everyone always ends up standing around in the kitchen.

Do you want nourishment or chaos from your kitchen? A pleasant, organized kitchen leads to less eating out, which in turn means better nutrition, less money spent on food, and more family together time. The kitchen should be a place where you want to spend time, a place where you take pleasure in preparing and eating food, a place that fosters eating as a communal activity. A place of growth and warmth. There is no other room in a home, however, that is expected to serve more purposes than the kitchen. This multipurpose chaos can cloud the kitchen's importance in the life and health of you and your family.

Kitchens can easily become collecting grounds for food "ideas" that never come to fruition: vegetables rot in refrigerator drawers; frozen vegetables fill up freezer doors; and pantries are stuffed with out-of-date soup and boxes of rice and cartons of oatmeal that we think we should eat but never manage to prepare. Drawers and cabinets are stuffed with second and third sets of dishes and specialty items, like fondue and serving dishes, that haven't seen the light of day since you stored them away after your wedding.

If your home is a reflection of who you are, then your kitchen is a reflection of the way you eat and the way you feel about food. You're not sure this is correct? Try an exercise with me.

Spend a few minutes walking around your kitchen and try to look at it as though seeing it for the first time. What do you feel when you walk into the room? What's the first thing that you notice? How do the countertops look? The sink? Open a few cupboards and drawers and get a sense of what is in them. Are they organized? Is it clear what each is used for? Take a look at what food you have in the kitchen. Does it look appetizing? Is most of it in packages? Is there much at all? Open the refrigerator. What do you see? What do you smell? What is your overall mood in this room? What is the most important function of this room?

Food? The family office? Homework and project central? Imagine meeting your spouse for the first time. Would you bring him or her home to eat a dinner prepared in this kitchen? Does your kitchen reflect the life you want? What does it say about you?

Dear Peter:

Often just the thought of sifting through the clutter on the countertop to make way for the pots and pans and the thought of clearing out the sink to cook a healthy meal left me with only one option: "Let's go out to eat!" We never sought a healthy meal in that mood. We wasted time and money eating many unhealthy calories.

When your house is clutter-free (which it is now, thanks to finishing your book, *It's All Too Much*), one can think clearly, and into the future, even though the future is only five hours away, about what to make for dinner, and when you have clean, clear countertops it makes you look forward to, rather than dread, cooking dinner!

Define your vision for the kitchen you want

Words that describe your ideal kitchen:

- _____

- _____

- _____

- _____

- _____

In my ideal kitchen, I would be able to:

_____

_____

In my ideal kitchen, my family would be able to:

_____

_____

For most of my clients, this is the first time they've really studied their kitchens. While they probably look at the kitchen every day and spend a great deal of time there, seeing it in a new light is revealing and often unsettling. The arrangement and state of your house — including your kitchen — has a direct impact on the rest of your life. This link, almost always overlooked, is one that I can't emphasize enough. In movies, the instruction "get your house in order" is what the concerned doctor always says to the patient who has just learned she has three months to live. It refers to the most important things one needs to do before dying, getting one's life in order. Why wait till you're on your deathbed to do it?

Your kitchen is the source of nutrition for your family — both in the narrow meaning of the food you eat, but also in a broader sense of providing part of the mood, attitude, motivation, and atmosphere of well-being that should be present in your household. Your kitchen is the place that feeds your household. It has to be part of the vision you have for the life you want and the home that is important to you. A key element in the recent renovation of my own home was the removal of a wall to open the kitchen space to the rest of the living area of the house. The ability to share meals with family and friends in one large, warm, welcoming space was critical to the design of our home and to what we felt to be most important in our lives: celebration, friendship, warmth, and sharing. Our kitchen makes a clear statement about our lives and our family. Does your own kitchen do the same?

The kitchen is the nerve center of any home. It is usually the first port of call when anyone comes into a home and often the place where most of the action takes place — hanging and chatting, cooking, eating, doing homework, or even paying the bills. It is where important things happen and it's those things you want to cultivate in your home — great meals prepared with ease, better nutrition for you and your family, pleasure in spending time in a welcoming environment, a desire for healthy food and so less inclination to grab takeout and, perhaps most important of all, the cultivation of a positive outlook for you and your family.

A kitchen for cooking

Why do you have a kitchen in your house?

Discover the truth about your kitchen

TRIGGERS THAT LEAD ME TO OVEREAT

My kitchen is a place where I/we:	True/False
1. Let mail or other junk pile up	
2. Watch TV	
3. Store food	
4. Hang out	
5. Do work/homework	
6. Prepare food	
7. Feed pets	
8. Keep lots of pots and pans and other kitchen supplies that we rarely use	
9. Eat dinner	
10. Dance the Texas two-step	

The primary purpose of the kitchen is nourishment. The way it is organized should make food preparation easy and pleasant. If you answered "true" to numbers 3 and 6 and "false" to everything else, you're in good shape. And if you also eat in the kitchen, number 9, at a nice, clean table, that's a fine use for the space, as well (we'll talk more about your dining table in the next section). If you didn't answer "true" to numbers 3 and 6, well, it's time to go out and buy a refrigerator and an oven!

Now, if you answered "true" to any additional kitchen activities, we need to do some thinking and prioritizing. It's plain and simple: Getting good food onto your table comes first. Anything that interferes with that should be moved out of the kitchen — even the two-stepping!

Survey the space that you have

Kitchens do not create themselves. While every house has a room where the food preparation, cooking, eating, and clean up take place, not every house has a well-functioning kitchen that attracts and nurtures people. That's where you come in!

First simply check out the different spaces in your kitchen — the cupboards, the areas you have to prepare food, the amount of countertop you have, storage areas, space for cleaning up, and the amount of room you have to move around. Survey what you have in order to get an idea of what is possible and what is reasonable for the space.

Take note of what the room is used for beyond the normal kitchen function — homework, school projects, bill paying, laundry folding. Make a list as long as you want to cover all the activities that go on in your kitchen. Once you have this list completed, and a sense of the space you have available, we can get to work.

Think of your kitchen in terms of zones

You have to strike a balance in your kitchen between the needs of everyone in your home and the recognition that this is the area intended to feed and nourish your family. We need to divide the kitchen into specific areas or "zones" to help organize and make the most use of the space. The zones related to food preparation and serving are the most important ones and after they are established you can create other zones — like areas for homework or hobbies or bill paying — if space permits. However, it is your nutritional needs that must always take priority in this room.

There are four main activity zones that

have to be established in any kitchen: the preparation area, the cooking center, the eating area (if you have one), and the cleanup area. If you don't have an eat-in kitchen, incorporate the dining room into your plan as your eating area. Keeping in mind the space you have, and the layout of your kitchen, decide where each of these areas of activity will be. Even though these areas may be obvious — for example, the cleanup zone is where the sink is located in the room — it's important to keep these specific areas in your mind as we move forward.

Look again at the space you have and decide what other zones or areas for specific activities you need and that the kitchen has room for. Now complete the list below, noting what is needed for each of those zones to work the way you want. I have given you some ideas to get you started. You may want to add more zones to meet your specific needs.

Break the kitchen into zones

ZONE	ITEMS NEEDED	
	My suggestions	**Your suggestions**
Preparation area	Cutting board Knives Mixing bowls	
Cooking center	Pots and pans Spices Utensils	
Eating area	Flatware Glasses Napkins	
Cleanup area	Drying rack Dishwashing liquid Sponge and scourer	
POSSIBLE ADDITIONAL ZONES		
Homework area	Construction paper Pens and pencils	
Bill paying area	Checkbook Stamps Pens	

You'll notice that I haven't included food storage, a key area in any kitchen. The pantry is so central to the smooth functioning of the kitchen and the well-being of your family that we're going to address it separately.

Identifying the items needed in each zone will help you as you move into the next phase.

GET YOUR KITCHEN'S WEIGHT UNDER CONTROL!

Kitchens attract a ton of useless but seemingly "must-have" gadgets and gizmos. Tune into late-night infomercials if you don't believe me! If you bought it over the phone after 8:00 p.m., chances are you don't need it. The first step to getting organized is to seriously pare down the amount of food, dishes, and appliances in your kitchen. Discard those items that have outlived their usefulness. Do you really need to keep that bread maker just because it was a Christmas present? It's taking up valuable counter space. And those specialty pots and pans, egg slicers, apple corers, melon ballers, and who knows what — do you really use them?

As terrifying as it might sound, what you need to do now is to help your kitchen shed some of those excess pounds that have accumulated over the years. Assess what you have in your kitchen and discard what is no longer necessary. Be brave — this is an important step in the process. Making your kitchen lighter is a step toward making yourself lighter. Cleaning out your kitchen is a two-part process: the Quick Purge and the Deep Clean. Be ruthless in the Quick Purge and, I promise, the Deep Clean will be easier.

Quick Purge and Deep Clean your kitchen

The Quick Purge

Start at one end of your kitchen and go through each cupboard and drawer quickly and efficiently. Pull anything out that you no longer use or need and also remove anything that doesn't belong in the kitchen — toys, crafting materials, car parts, musical instruments. You get the idea. Anything that isn't used for food preparation, storing, serving, or cleanup has to go. Pull out the duplicates of items you have and decide which is the better one to keep. If it's broken — toss it. If it's stained or chipped beyond use — throw it out. If you don't like it — get rid of it. The goal here is to quickly remove those items that you definitely don't want, need, or use. It shouldn't take much thought or emotional energy to get this done. The secret is to move as quickly as you can. Place all these items on the counter or floor or even in a wheelbarrow parked in the kitchen if that works for you — just get it done! Then, just as quickly, get all the items you no longer need out of your kitchen. Remember that the more space you clear at this stage, the less work you'll have to do in the next round.

The Deep Clean

Already you should notice a difference in the look and feel of your kitchen. Simply decluttering, without any organizing, opens up more space than most people can imagine. Now, look again at the zones or activity centers you listed in the table (see pages 114–115). You now need to move logically through your kitchen and remove everything from every cupboard — you can do the drawers in the same way later. (Note: You can break up this Deep Clean over time. Clear out one drawer or cabinet each evening instead of watching TV. You may even find yourself so focused on that goal that you end up snacking less.)

As you move through the space considering whether to keep or discard each item in your kitchen, ask yourself these simple questions:

1. Have I used this in the last twelve months (six months if you're fearless!)?

2. Do I enjoy using this kitchen tool/ appliance?
3. Does this make food preparation easier or more efficient?
4. Is this easy to clean?
5. Do I have all the pieces for this?
6. Do I want this in my kitchen?

If the answer to any of these questions is no, then that item has no place in your kitchen — it has to go. I constantly say that the only items in your home should be things that you love and that you use. It's the same principle in the kitchen.

If you decide that an item should stay, determine in which zone in your kitchen you will use it and place it in an area on your kitchen counter or table with other similar items. It might help to make signs for each zone as temporary labels to keep track of what goes where. Be ruthless. Stripping away this excess "fat" from your kitchen is as important as the weight you wish to strip away from your hips.

At the end of the process discard, donate, or dig a hole in the backyard to bury the things that no longer belong in your kitchen so that they don't get a chance to come back into the house. Trust me, if you leave them lying around, the temptation to sneak them into a drawer or cupboard somewhere will be too great! Finally, take this opportunity to wipe down shelves and the inside of cupboards and drawers.

You should now have only those things that you need, use, and take pleasure in. Return them to your kitchen cupboards.

Dear Peter:

About a year ago, I completely decluttered my kitchen and I was so consumed by the task that I didn't focus on food. I actually began to do a sort of "fast" in a natural sort of way. I was performing a cleanse on my kitchen and a simultaneous cleanse of my body. Normally, I am obsessed with food so this seemed unusual to me. At this point, I carry about ten to fifteend pounds more than feels comfortable to me, and in the same way my house is cluttered with extra "fat." I thought that I had some sort of organizational disability, but now I think that my clutter protects me in some way (the same way that a little tire of fat around the middle can protect you). Clutter is a way of sabotaging my life in the same way that gaining weight makes me feel helpless and hopeless about my body.

Get help

If you don't live alone, I see no reason why you should do all the purging alone. Unless, of course, it's *your* mess, in which case you should stop complaining and get to work. But taking the time to clean out your kitchen and pantry as a family is a great opportunity to open the lines of communication. Start in the morning with full stomachs all around, and have lunch — sandwiches or a salad — ready in advance. You don't want the day to devolve into a snackfest. Now get to work.

The kitchen is really easy to divide up. Give your partner and children tasks that make sense for their age and ability. A small child can be enlisted to take everything out of the lower shelves in the pantry (assuming, of course, that these shelves aren't loaded with toxic cleaning agents and sharp knives). A preteen can clean out the refrigerator. Even a teen can be persuaded to identify pots, pans, and kitchen gizmos that you never use. As you clean together, you may find yourselves sharing memories of holidays past, or talking about the fondue parties you always thought you'd have some day. Make this a day when, without getting into any fights, your husband can finally admit that he hates the way you cook rice or your wife can confess that she's glad you do the dishes, but she always washes the pots again after you've done them.

Zoning Out

Once you've completed your Quick Purge and Deep Clean, it's time to get your kitchen in order and put your zones into action.

Work around the "magic triangle"

As you decide which areas represent your specific zones, and where things belong, keep in mind what is often referred to as the "magic triangle." Think of the area formed by your sink, refrigerator, and oven or stove top as the magic triangle of your kitchen. This triangle is sacred ground — the focus of food preparation, cleanup, and serving. Anything that is central to your daily food preparation (pots, wooden spoons, food storage bags, everyday dishes, etc.) should be located in or on the sides of this imaginary triangle. Nothing else should be in this area. One step out of the triangle are all of those things that you use regularly, but infrequently, in your kitchen: food processor, mixer, specialty pots. One step farther is stuff you seldom use: bread maker, turkey pan, holiday cookie cutters. Systematically begin placing items into their designated zone or area. Be smart and place heavier, less frequently used items relatively low in cupboards and the lighter, less-used items higher but still within easy reach. By organizing your kitchen in this way, you will find yourself moving efficiently in the space with minimum movement for maximum return. By having important and frequently used items close, you will save an enormous amount of time and energy in your kitchen. Suddenly it will be both a breeze and a pleasure to work in the space.

Dear Peter:

If I got rid of the clutter in my kitchen and fridge, I would be able to easily find what I needed to prepare healthier meals. It's at least 60 percent of the battle. Having cleaned off counters/workspaces is heaven. The more space I have, the more I tend to prepare meals that require more (and usually better) ingredients. The less workspace I have, the more I tend to prepare less "complicated" meals (because I have nowhere to put the ingredients).

Whether it's plates, pots and pans, or food items, be sure to keep similar items together and organized in each zone. Following this rule will also save time and money as you can quickly and easily see what items you already have. When it comes to foodstuffs, you can quickly take stock of what you have and avoid overpurchasing.

MAGIC TRIANGLE CHEAT SHEET

Most people don't organize their kitchens. They just unpack when they move in and never change where things go. It's time for a rethink. (And while you make changes, you'll have a chance to clean out some of those drawers that never get cleaned.)

Items related to food storage go near the refrigerator. Think: containers, clips, foil, and plastic bags.

Items related to food preparation go near the sink. Think: knives, cutting boards, and colanders.

Items related to cooking (and baking) go near the stove or cooktop. Think: pots, pans, and cooking utensils.

Also included in the magic triangle are everyday dishes.

One step outside the triangle: Items you use regularly, but infrequently. Think: food processor, mixer, and specialty pots.

One step farther (or on a high shelf out of reach): Items you rarely use. Think: bread maker, turkey pan, holiday cookie cutters.

Keep flat surfaces clear

After establishing zones, keeping flat surfaces clear is perhaps the single most important thing to keep in mind for your kitchen — as it is for any room in the house. A clear countertop makes any kitchen look more organized and feel more welcoming. Plus it's definitely easier to clean. It encourages people to gather and makes food preparation something that can be enjoyed. Once the flat surfaces start to disappear under clutter, you lose your motivation to keep the area organized. Then the area starts to attract dust and dirt, further compounding the clutter problem. Consider flat surfaces your preparation area — not your storage area!

Cookbooks and recipes

If you already have cookbooks and recipes taking up space in your kitchen, purge any that you never use and never will. Find an inexpensive scrapbook or file to hold all of those fantastic recipes you find in magazines, are given by friends, or that your grandmother left to you. Keep the scrapbook with other cookbooks in a central place in your kitchen. Go through your cookbooks and discard any you haven't opened in a year. If, by chance, you do one day need a recipe for Bavarian Apple Strudel Custard Cake there is always the Internet.

A REFRIGERATOR WITH A VIEW

The refrigerator is the most important part of the magic triangle. This is where you store the foods you plan to eat in the next few days. What do you want from your refrigerator? What it should be is a place to temporarily store healthy foods for your family. What it should *not* be is a place where you stand, with the door open, gazing at a crowded jumble of assorted foods, trying to figure out how in the world you can possibly combine them to make a meal. In Chapter 6 we're going to make a shopping list and go to the store together, but let's start talking in general terms about what you should have in your refrigerator.

Food in the refrigerator should be food with a plan. Anything that belongs in the refrigerator has an expiration date. This means that it will go bad. So if you don't have an immediate plan to use something, get rid of it. Remember, the point here isn't to hold on to foods because you might have a use for them someday. Band-Aids are something it's good to have on hand in case of an emergency, food is not (other than, say, earthquake survival food). It makes no sense to say, "You never know when you might need to eat." You need to eat every day! Several times a day! It also doesn't make sense to say, "You never know when you might get home late and have to make dinner in a rush." You know that happens to you. You know about how often it happens. It should be part of your plan when you shop for food.

Clean your refrigerator every week, preferably right before you go shopping. Throw away food that's gone bad. Then, when you come home from the grocery store, organize your food in a logical way. As you put in the new foods, move the older foods to the front so they get used up first. If you have the space, devote one drawer to vegetables, one to fruit, and one to meats. Use a smaller drawer for cheese or snacks. Keep like items together — all dairy products huddle on one shelf. All snacks cluster together. All prepared foods stack neatly. If you have time, do yourself a favor and wash and dry vegetables and fruits that can handle it (yes: grapes; no:

berries) before putting them away so that they're ready to go when you want to use them.

Fruits and Vegetables

If you regularly find yourself throwing away bruised pears and limp greens, don't accept this as a fact of life. The problem may not be that you bought too much. Chances are that when you were in the grocery store, you were imagining healthy, balanced, colorful meals and snacks with food from all the food groups. You bought a reasonable amount of fruit and vegetables, brought them home, and promptly gravitated to cookies. Rotten fruit and vegetables mean you didn't have a plan, so you've been eating too much easy food.

Condiments

Mustard, jelly, salad dressing, pickles . . . what is all that stuff that spends eternity languishing in the door of your refrigerator? Every few months, take a look at those condiments. Make sure they have plenty of room and don't overflow beyond the door. The door is the only place where condiments are allowed. Throw away those jars you're unlikely to open again. And, please, remember that nothing lasts forever. Try taping the lid shut, write the date on the tape and check it three months later. Get rid of everything that still has tape holding it closed.

Why bother?

If all this seems like a lot of work, you're right! It is. Success doesn't come without some personal investment. We're investing in your life here! However, if you're serious about losing weight and taking a healthier approach to life, an organized, clean kitchen is key to making it work. You know how little incentive there is to work in a kitchen that is cluttered, disorganized, and in which it's hard to move around. Every aspect of preparing a meal in a chaotic kitchen takes more time and more effort, but if you don't do the work now to organize, all too soon you'll find yourself settling for the easy option — takeout. Who needs the aggravation when you can pick up the phone and order an extralarge pepperoni pizza and (because you're so weight conscious) a large diet soda! Don't sabotage yourself. Clear out the excess now so you don't succumb to temptation later!

Cupboards and drawers

The easier it is to find things in your kitchen,

the more pleasant your whole food experience will be. Let's tour some typical trouble spots.

Pots and pans

Pots and pans are awkward and hard to store. Ceiling racks or corner cupboards with rotating trays help, but if you don't have those options, pare down your collection to the minimum. Give away pots you don't use. Store big pots that you only use occasionally farther from the magic triangle.

Utensils

Use dividers in your utensil drawer. Sorting forks and spoons is a great way for young children to help unload the dishwasher. If you have one big drawer for all your cooking tools, go through it regularly. Get rid of those strange gizmos that you never use. And — please! — don't mix sharp knives or scissors with other utensils. Keep knives easily accessible in your food preparation area.

Food storage containers

Try sealing up each of your plastic containers with a bit of masking tape. As you use them, you'll take off the tape. After a month or two, get rid of all the containers that are still taped shut. Also, don't overheat or overuse plastic containers. Plastic is only tested for the manufacturer's intended use. If you treat it differently, you risk plastic compounds wandering into your food. Not a pleasant thought.

Junk

More than anything, I want you to rid your kitchen of junk. Don't let mail pile up. Keep flat surfaces clear. Don't let the kitchen be a catchall for things that don't have a place in your home. Everything should have a place in your home that makes sense for where and how you use it. No junk drawer full of odds and ends and bits of broken toys. No. Junk.

A PANTRY WITH A PURPOSE

Pantries are harder to manage than refrigerators. Why? Our pantries are usually chock full of foods that we buy because they look good, or because they seem like good foods to have on hand, or because they're on sale. They're sort of like clothes closets — full of impulse purchases and sale mistakes. Instead of being the place your food goes to expire, make your pantry a staging area for healthy living. If you're going to experiment by buying new things, make sure you have a recipe and a plan for the whole meal you want to cook. The same goes for sale items. Getting a good price on that box of Arborio rice means nothing if you haven't the first clue about how to prepare risotto.

Dear Peter:

Your pantry should be neat and organized, with infrequently used items less accessible and daily items up front.

If my pantry is organized I can see what foods I have and can gather things to make healthy meals, rather than run out to the grocery store to get the "missing" ingredient. Then dinner is late and I am hungry and more apt to grab a few quick — and not the most healthy — things to eat along the way.

Take everything out and clean

That's right, pull every single box out of the pantry. This will give you a great opportunity to clean up all the nuts and bits of cereal that have escaped and are roaming freely among the bags and boxes.

Toss

Get rid of everything that's stale, expired, or infested (it happens). Now look at what you've got left. You're only going to put back those boxes that look like old friends because you've finished and repurchased them so many times. Anything else has to go.

Shop for your pantry

We're going to make our shopping lists in the next chapter, but let's talk about how your pantry should work. I tell people that you can't have more books than you have room on your bookshelves, and the same logic applies to all other shelves, cupboards, and drawers in your home. If you overstuff your pantry, you won't use it effectively. Before you go shopping, compare your pantry to your shopping list. Make sure you haven't listed items you already have enough of. A lot of pantry purchases are impulse buys. You pick up yet another box of instant oatmeal because it seems like something you might need, only to come home and find you already have three boxes. This is why you must make a list before you shop and stick to it. If you have limited room in your pantry (and who doesn't?), you need to think carefully before you buy anything. If you only use flour occasionally, don't buy a five-pound bag. Resist the great price on the restaurant-size jar of mayonnaise. You only need enough tomato sauce for one week —

you can always buy more. Let me say that again: "Enough" is a week's supply. You're not going into hibernation for winter.

When you shop for your pantry, be mindful of clutter foods. Like the boxes full of who-knows-what filling your basement or garage, clutter foods are foods that you think you should have in your house, but don't really eat. Let's examine some of the foods that take up room in our cupboards.

Aspirational Foods

Aspirational foods are foods that you buy with the hope that you'll magically turn into a person you're not. They're baking goods for the person who never bakes. They're gourmet spices for a frozen-food junkie. They're Tibetan *goji* berries with magical antioxidant qualities when you're fantasizing that one little food can serve all your nutritional needs. I'm all for adventure and experimentation, but if you're never going to canoe down the Rio Grande, there's no point in storing that boat in your garage. And if the *goji* berry moment has passed? Let it go.

Entertainment Foods

You read in some magazine once that every good hostess should always have a few key items on hand for spontaneous entertaining. Then you promptly went out and bought a jar of olives, several boxes of crackers, some quince paste or exotic honey, and a few other obscure pantry items. It felt good to know that if you ran into someone on the street you could say, "Come on in for a glass of wine." You were so organized and ready! Yeah, that was four years and two apartments ago, and you've packed up and moved the margarita mix and salt from one pantry to the next. Let's face it, you're either antisocial, or when you entertain you always end up shopping for fresh ingredients. No matter how you slice it, those olives have got to go.

Security Foods

Do you eat healthy meals for breakfast, lunch, and dinner, but keep a secret stash of the junk food that you truly love in your pantry? You try to eat well, but sometimes you just want a good old box of macaroni and orange-powdered "cheese." Or a giant bag of potato chips. Maybe it just makes you feel better to know that should you suffer a major craving and require an instant chocolate fix, the pantry has a limitless supply of semisweet chocolate chips that you have no intention of using to make cookies.

You think these foods make you feel more secure — like you don't have to binge because you know you could have them whenever you want. But your mac 'n' cheese is deceiving you. It's not there for a rainy day. It's there to be eaten as dinner. Or a snack. Whenever you're disorganized and prone to reaching for the easiest fix. These aren't security foods. They are naughty foods (if they can even be called food), and they don't belong in your pantry. Bye-bye!

Emergency Food

Yes, I know all those emergency preparedness checklists that they hand out at your local street fair have lists of all the nonperishable cans and jars of food and water that you should have on hand in case of global thermonuclear war. Here's all I have to say on the matter: Buying emergency foods is like buying insurance — you hope you never have to use them. All of your emergency supplies should be in an out-of-the-way place like the basement, the garage, a storage closet, or the far back of your pantry (if it's particularly large). The only exception to this is if you're organized enough to consume your emergency food supplies over time, rotating in fresher cans and jars. Hats off to you if you're actually pulling that off. You're one in a million.

Organize your pantry

You've purged your pantry of foods you don't eat. Now that you have a nice, clean cupboard with plenty of space, it's time to bring order to the foods you're storing.

Prioritize. As you put things away, prioritize them. Foods you use every day or quite often, like cereals or your favorite tea, should be on the shelf that is most accessible for you.

Group like things together. All the cereals should be together. All the nuts in one place.

178

Keeping like things together makes them easier to find and helps prevent duplicate purchases. If space is an issue and you need to use the full depth of your cupboard, be sure to put tall things in back and short things in front.

Make use of vertical space. If your shelves are too far apart you can buy inserts that add an extra shelf or racks that hang from the back of the pantry door. Add sliding shelves to maximize depth. If your storage is high, find an attractive stepladder that you don't mind having around your kitchen. A whole extra level of storage will suddenly be accessible.

Decant. Transfer foods that come in messy packaging into clear containers. Also decant if you have bug problems. Some containers dispense food at the bottom, so if you refill before the container is empty you'll still be using the oldest food first.

Physical upgrades

It always helps to have a bright, clear pantry so foods don't disappear into dark corners. A fresh coat of white paint and better lighting are a great way to make a fresh start. Also, invest in a spice rack that really works well for your space. If one fits over the back of your pantry door, it's a great way to keep spices visible and out of the way. A lazy Susan is also a good option for spices or other small pantry items.

A commitment to your kitchen is a commitment to yourself and the process to improve every aspect of your life. Enjoying your food starts with feeling happy in your kitchen. And if you don't enjoy your food, you'll never be happy with your body. It's that simple. Once your kitchen is clutter-free, it's time to fill it with well-chosen food.

CHECKLIST FOR CHAPTER FIVE

- ❏ Start with a decluttered home.
- ❏ Define your vision for your kitchen.
- ❏ Discover the truth about your kitchen.
- ❏ Divide the kitchen into zones.
- ❏ Quick Purge and Deep Clean your kitchen.
- ❏ Rethink the pantry.

Six:
The Food You Stock

Filling Your Kitchen
and Your Stomach

By now you have a clear vision of the life you want for yourself. You could easily tell me what that life looks like and how it is different from the life you are living now. Your home is clutter-free. The things you own, value, and honor are appropriately used or displayed. Your organized home is a reflection of the life you are creating for yourself every day — calm, ordered, and as stress-free as any of us can be with our busy lives and frequently crazy schedules.

Your kitchen — the room that nourishes and sustains your family — is a place that you enjoy using and spending time in. It's a room that creates a sense of harmony and relaxation. With little effort you can easily find what you need in your kitchen, pantry, and refrigerator.

If you don't have the right foundation for

moving forward, then you have work to do. Unless a clutter-free and organized space is your starting point, you are guaranteed failure. That may sound harsh, but it's really that simple. I am hoping that by now you can see the way this process is working. We started with the big picture — your life vision — and, using that as the foundation, have worked to create the spaces that support and encourage you to reach your goals of happiness — your home, your kitchen, and even your pantry and refrigerator! I hope that through the process of decluttering your home you have noticed some interesting secondary effects. Less stress, increased focus, higher motivation, more inner peace, and less time eating foods that are unhealthy choices for you. You have opened and lightened your physical space and are now making inroads by addressing the weight issues that bother you. Now it's time to plan what you eat. And I don't use the words "time" and "plan" lightly.

PLAN YOUR DAY, PLAN YOUR TIME, PLAN YOUR LIFE

Although it might not always feel that way, you control your life. You make the decisions about what you do, when you do it, and with whom. Sure, there are some things that are beyond our control, like the weather. But when it rains, you decide if you want to wear a cheerful raincoat, forgo the umbrella to enjoy an invigorating soak, or grumble and moan your way through a gray, dreary day. You are the boss of your life and I want *you* to govern with the principles of balance, proportion, and logic. Don't let emotions drive your actions or what you do will be subject to mood and whim. Follow the *plan,* not the *feelings.* Balance your obligations with your priorities. Commit your time in proportion to your goals. Make logical, conscious choices. Planning is not a gratuitous activity that you should do to prove to the world how on top of things you are. Planning means you know what you want from your life and you're determined to follow the path you've designed to get there. If you're not driving your life, who is?

QUIZ

Are You a Planner?

Answer the following "true" or "false":

1. I keep a calendar with all my appointments.
2. I'm rarely late.

3. I do my laundry regularly enough that I never run out of underwear.
4. I've run out of gas less than three times in my life.
5. I return phone calls (at least the ones I want to return) within forty-eight hours.
6. I never pay late fees on bills.
7. If older than thirty, I've prepared my will and advanced health care directives, and I have life and health insurance.
8. If I were planning a wedding, I'd have a spreadsheet with every key element scheduled.
9. If someone asked me for my most recent financial statements I'd be able to pull them out without much fuss.
10. In my home, I know where almost everything is.
11. I make plans for holidays or family members'/friends' birthdays well ahead of time.
12. I'd describe my work situation as "under control."
13. I exercise at least three days per week.
14. I usually prepare a shopping list when I go to the grocery store.

15. I know at least a day in advance what I'm doing for the next day's meals.
16. I don't rush my children out the door. If it takes ten minutes for them to tie their shoes, so be it.
17. I never forget an important birthday or anniversary.
18. I get my hair cut on a regular schedule.

This questionnaire covers the major organizational points of our lives. I'm not going to grade you on your answers to this quiz. But I do want you to look at your responses.

Score yourself

If almost all your answers were "true":
You're an organized person. Your life is under control. You're probably successful and thriving in your career. Anyone who met you would think, Here's a responsible, together person. That's great. But now you need to look at the few questions to which your response was "false." Why are these areas different for you? Why are you resistant to addressing these critical parts of your life? If you answered "true" to everything except

the last two or three questions, about exercising and preparing food, you're not alone. For a surprising number of people, their own bodies are the last frontier. We take our health for granted. Eating can be an emotional issue. Most of us develop our work and home organization routines as adults, but our bad health habits start in childhood and are harder to break. That's why you're here, to bring your body up to the level of the rest of your life. You'll be as successful at this as you are at everything else. You just have to work on it.

If almost all your answers were "false":

Life can be overwhelming. Sometimes we have to focus so hard on one element of our lives — work, relationships, family, emotional well-being — that it's hard to keep the rest in balance. My acquaintance Andrew, an architect, runs his own small firm. He also has a wife and two young children. He has very little free time and chooses to spend it reading to his children before bed every night because for him that's more important than opening the mail, much less paying the bills. He says there just isn't enough time in the day and he has to prioritize. This is understandable as a temporary situation, but when things pile up exponentially it gets hard to dig out. Now that his children are seven and eight, years of neglect have led to insurmountable clutter in his house. Andrew says he'll deal with it when his kids are in college. We'll see. If Andrew were my client, I'd ask him to sacrifice one night a week of reading to the children. He'd explain to them that though it is important to him, he also wants them to have a home that is ordered and he wants the family finances to be organized. I'd have him enlist the children in their own projects on the same evening. I'm sure their reading skills wouldn't suffer, and they'd learn some valuable skills for the future.

If you live in a state of general disorder, you need to deal with that. Stop buying diet books and fretting about your figure. Focus on getting rid of the clutter and organizing your life, and you'll find that weight loss follows.

If your answers were half "true," half "false":

We're all human, nobody's perfect, etc., etc. What I want you to do is to look down the list of questions and use your answers to evaluate what your priorities are. If a stranger looked at your quiz, what areas of your life would he identify as your priorities? Work? Finances? The household? And *are* those things most important to you? Is your behavior in line with what is most important

187

to you? Because if your energy is going toward the wrong end, no wonder you feel out of control. No wonder you're not as happy as you could be. You need to focus on what matters the most.

You picked up this book because your body and health are important to you. But if they're a priority, are you spending your time efficiently — that is, are you seeing results? Are you spending hours at the gym for months on end without dropping a pound? Are you constantly worrying about what you eat but still making bad choices? You need a new approach. A new plan.

FOOD-CLUTTER PRINCIPLE

If it isn't healthy, colorful, and part of your meal plan, don't eat it. It's junk.

Plan your meals

Now we get to the tricky part. What should you actually be eating? It may surprise you to find that I am not going to provide you with menus and sample meals. That's not my area of expertise, nor do I think it's what you need. There are a million cookbooks that describe healthy meals. You don't need me to tell you that salad is good for you, or to eat vegetables and fruits of all different (natural) colors, or to eat lean protein. Nor do you need me to tell you to eat whole grains and low-fat dairy, to drink water rather than soda. You already know that pigging out is bad, and that you should be eating reasonably sized meals. Eat regularly, eat better, and eat less. If your fat is an issue for you, chances are you know more about food than I ever will. You already know what you should be eating, what your meals should look like, and what it is you should be avoiding — how can you not? You've heard these "secrets" from every diet book that's failed you. The focus here is not on the foods you should be eating, but on finding the motivation, commitment, and ability to plan to eat the foods that are best for you. It's not about the diet. It's about the decision.

As I have found when helping people declutter and organize their homes, there is a compass within you that will point you in the right direction. Unless you've just arrived from another planet, I suspect that you are already food literate and know what foods are nutritious. Not tasteless — nutritious. Do you know what is in the food that goes into your mouth? Have you checked the label on the packaged food you have for dinner? You wouldn't think of swallowing a test tube of propylene glycol alginate or disodium guanylate, yet there's no problem if your salad dressing is laced with it. Do you eat healthy food at meals and chips or candy for snacks? Do you indulge in dessert . . . after every meal? Or are your meals themselves loaded with fat or salt? Are they unbalanced? Is all the food on your plate just varying shades of brown? Eating the foods you already know are good for you in the right portions will help you lose weight without cramping your style. Let's do a simple exercise to see how what you know stacks up against what you eat. Complete as fully and honestly as you can the following table:

ACTIVITY	
Make a truthful list of what you know	
WHAT I KNOW ABOUT THE FOOD I EAT	
Foods I eat and love that are good for me:	
Foods I eat and love that are not good for me:	

Make a truthful list of what you know

WHAT I KNOW ABOUT THE FOOD I EAT

Foods I eat too little of:	
Foods I eat too much of:	
Foods in my home right now that help create the life and body I want:	
Foods in my home right now that sabotage the life and body I want:	

Stop for a moment and look closely at the lists you've composed. If you ever needed evidence that you don't need me to tell you what you need to eat, it's right there in front of you. You are not a stupid person. We both know that you are perfectly aware of what you should and should not be eating. So enough of the charts and tables and portion measuring devices that clutter your life. These things are usually distractions that just add stress and pressure. While they may give a temporary sense of control, they are not what is needed to create the permanent change you are seeking in your life.

Look into yourself. I honestly believe that you have the knowledge, the good sense, and the instinct to know what is best for your body, your health, and your happiness in the life you are creating for yourself. That said, I'm here to give you a firm push in the right direction. Take a deep breath, keep the lists you've just completed handy, and let's go.

WHAT WORKS AND WHAT DOESN'T

You have already started thinking about the food choices that you make: what contributes to a healthier you and what sabotages that effort. Just the act of thinking through and writing down what you know about the foods you eat is an important start. The next step builds on the first.

Identify your healthier choices

When we cleaned up your kitchen, we talked about function. I asked you to get rid of anything that wasn't being used or treated with respect. Now we're going to do the same with food. Look at the foods on your list on pages 190–191. Which are the healthier choices? Using these as starter ideas, fill in the center column in the chart below. Then quickly jot down any ideas you have for food or meals that you can add to your list of healthy favorites. These are the choices you can see yourself making as you move to a healthier, more positive place.

YOUR HEALTHIER CHOICES CHART		
Meals	Starter ideas	Healthier foods or meals
Breakfast		
Lunch		
Dinner		
Snacks		

Here's how one client filled out this chart:

YOUR HEALTHIER CHOICES CHART		
Meals	**Starter ideas**	**Healthier foods or meals**
Breakfast	*Cereal, yogurt*	*Egg-white scramble*
Lunch	*Turkey sandwich*	*Soup and salad*
Dinner	*Chicken stir-fry*	*Roast chicken with vegetables*
Snacks	*Protein bar*	*Fruit, nuts, and hummus*

Fill out the columns as best you can. You'll be surprised at how many options you'll be able to imagine yourself eating and enjoying.

FRESH START — IN AT THE DEEP END

Lives are busy. Time always seems short. Everything is so complicated. Each day is made up of obligations, desires, habits, and mistakes, all spun into a fast-paced whir. So how are you supposed to reset your priorities? Where do you begin? Right here, with a Fresh Start. It's tough, it's radical, but it's necessary to move you to the next level.

Dear Peter:

I want the clutter out of my house and I want my extra pounds gone. I feel like if I don't do this for myself, I will never be happy with anything. I must do it and I'm determined to do it. My deadline to start is the beginning of the next school year in late August. Vacations will be over, my work schedule will loosen a bit, and I'll have no more excuses. Yippee! I'm excited to begin!

If we're going to make this work I'll need a half to a full day of your time. Don't have the time? Really? What is most important to you? What brings you closer to the life you want to live? Yes, I thought so. Forget the excuses. Let's get to it.

1. Set aside a day.

Remember what I said about making the time? This is your commitment to the life you want to live. What is it worth to you? What better plan did you have for today? There is no greater investment you can make than time devoted to creating the life you want.

2. Write down a week of ideal meals and snacks.

I'm not a food expert, and you don't have to be, either. Let's demystify this whole hoo-ha about what you should eat right here and now. Take five minutes and write down a quick and dirty meal plan for a week. Keep in mind what you know about the foods you should and shouldn't be eating. Take a few moments to look at the list you made a little earlier and just make it up. Imagine what a healthy, fit you would eat. I have absolutely no doubt that you can do it. Just put down a few clear, healthy choices. I don't care so much what your plan says, and nobody's going to grade your work. Here, I'll give you an example. This is what my client Lynne put down for her Fresh Start:

Meal	Monday	Tuesday	Wednesday	Thursday	Friday	Saturday	Sunday
Breakfast	Oatmeal	Yogurt with fruit and whole-grain toast	Egg-white omelet and whole-grain toast	Protein smoothie	Oatmeal	Yogurt with fruit and whole-grain toast	Egg-white scramble
Snack	Carrot sticks and nuts	Apple with a little cheese	Broccoli and hummus	Cottage cheese and berries	Stick of string cheese and nuts	Grapes and a little cheese	Bowl of multigrain cereal
Lunch	Turkey breast sandwich on multigrain bread	Salad, dressing on side	Soup and half tuna sandwich on rye	Salad, dressing on side	California roll and seaweed salad	Turkey breast sandwich on multigrain bread	Salad, dressing on side
Snack	Yogurt	Yogurt	Yogurt	Yogurt	Yogurt	Yogurt	Yogurt
Dinner	Chicken breast, asparagus, brown rice	Salmon, avocado, mango	Tofu stir-fry with vegetables	Veggie burger	Soup and salad	Pork chop, green beans, wild rice	White fish with vegetable

So you get the idea. Imagine healthy choices that you can see yourself eating — this is not a life sentence, it's just a week! Give it a shot.

Create a menu for next week

Meal	Monday	Tuesday	Wednesday	Thursday	Friday	Saturday	Sunday
Breakfast							
Snack							
Lunch							
Snack							
Dinner							

Like I said, it's not rocket science. The process is the same if you live in fast-food heaven or on a remote island. Write it down quickly and without overthinking it. What's important is that you get something down that you feel will work for you.

3. Get rid of all the food that's not part of your new eating plan.

I want you to get rid of everything else in your kitchen that isn't either on the menu plan you just completed or listed in the table of healthier choices you completed a little earlier. Yep — you heard me. All other food has to go. What? Why? No way! Stop the yelling for just a moment and listen to me. I want you to have a true fresh start.

Now you need to break old habits, and even though you have decluttered your kitchen and pantry and refrigerator, I'll bet those old habits are still ensconced in big and little ways in your home. Look again at the food that's still in your refrigerator and pantry. Be honest — does everything in those spaces speak to the life we are working to create for you? You need to start again. Old habits die hard. It's time to purge them for good. You're at a key turning point here. Dive in at the deep end. Commit or not — your call.

Ready? Let's do it.

4. A practical exception.

If you have a family or roommates and are embarking on this plan alone, removing their food from the house is not recommended. Try assigning space in your refrigerator or shelves in your pantry so that you stay away from others' food. Don't sneak their food. Who are you hiding from? Who are you cheating? Remember: You're doing this for yourself.

Get rid of any "Yesterday" foods in your home

Go through the refrigerator and the pantry. Make two piles, "The New Me" and "Yesterday."

THE NEW ME — what stays:

- Foods that appear on your Fresh Start menu or on your Healthier Choices chart.
- Foods belonging to someone else in the house that you know you won't touch.
- Tea and coffee.
- Condiments.

Work sensibly as you go through the food

that stays and goes. You probably have not listed cooking oil, condiments, and spices, for example, as part of your "New Me" items. Provided they are not past their use-by date, they can stay. Same goes for baking items if they're regularly used.

Keep the foods in your kitchen that you want to stay in your diet and on your menu. These are the foods you should be eating more often (assuming you have any of those in your kitchen!), foods that you love, that are good for you, and, most important, foods that help you create the body and the life you want. This is your plan, your kitchen, and your food, so use your common sense here. Don't obsess about individual items. If you're not sure whether to keep something, do what I advise my clients to do when they are decluttering their houses and can't decide if something should stay or go. Ask yourself: "Does this help me achieve the life I want for myself?"

If it does, keep it. If not, what's it doing in your home?

YESTERDAY — what goes:

- Frozen prepackaged meals masquerading as friends — you're not doing that anymore.

- ■ Fantasy foods — healthy or not, these are foods you had big dreams of preparing once upon a time but never have. If they're not on your Fresh Start menu or part of your Healthier Choices chart, they have to go.
- ■ Dry rice and pasta — they seem practical and useful, but if these items are not on your Fresh Start menu, they have to go.
- ■ Emergency foods — store enough emergency supplies for your family in a place separate from your pantry. Your pantry should only have foods that you are actively using.
- ■ High-calorie, nutritionally void, food-like items — cookies, chips, sweet snacks. It's hard, but you knew this was coming; now say good-bye.

You'll notice that I'm not being specific about what foods you can keep and what has to go. When it comes to healthier living one size doesn't fit all. We are individuals, and you need to make a commitment to decisions that work for you. Stop and reflect on what you *know* does not belong in your pantry and refrigerator — if it is part of the way you used to think of yourself, if it doesn't move you closer to the best you can be, why would you keep it anywhere close?

Look at the "Yesterday" pile. What you are looking at is not food — don't think of it like that. What you have before you is clutter that you have brought into your home. It is no different from the other household clutter that paralyzes and overwhelms and depresses you. Just like the stuff you've cleared from your home, this is the clutter you are clearing from your kitchen, your meals, your diet, and, ultimately, your life.

Look at the chart on pages 190–191 you filled out, which shows what you know about the foods you eat. See the foods you eat a lot of that aren't good for you? See the foods you eat too much of? As you move them to the "Yesterday" pile, take note of these foods. Wave good-bye and good riddance. You have just made a huge step toward conquering your fat. Again, it's a mistake to think of what you are discarding as food — it's not. With every item that you have chosen to remove from your kitchen, you are removing a hurdle — a hurdle that you put between yourself and your ideal body. A hurdle that you no longer have to struggle over to get to the life you want.

Now here's the hard part. Get rid of the "Yesterday" pile immediately!

You're horrified. What a waste of perfectly

good food! I didn't say anything about wasting it. Just get rid of it. Donate it to a charity. Give it to a friend. Have a free-food party. I don't care what you do, just get it out of the house immediately. Yes, I know it's money down the drain. But what does it cost you to keep these foods? If you don't start now, when will you start? What will tomorrow's excuse be? How much is your health and happiness worth? Because that's what being fat is costing you.

5. Buy the ingredients you need for your Fresh Start menu of meals.

I want you to do this in one single trip to one single grocery store. Go to the store with a list. Buy everything on that list, no more, no less. Try to buy in quantities that you think will last one week. Be aware of what you buy. As you carry your groceries into the house, feel their weight in your arms. Think about the number and weight of those bags. That's how much food you (or you and your family) plan to consume in a single week. Think of what this food and this shopping trip represent. There is nothing in those bags except items that are part of the life you want.

When you come home, as you unpack, look at the foods that you've purchased and imagine them going into your body. Are they wholesome and colorful? Would you feed them to a loved one? This is sustenance. This is life. Start to close the distance between yourself and what goes into your body.

Done? Good. Now we have one week where you know exactly what you're going to eat. It's a good thing, too, because you're going to be very busy.

FOOD-CLUTTER PRINCIPLE

Taking time to think out your meals teaches you how to verbalize what's important to you and to make choices based on those priorities.

PLANNING MEALS: NEXT WEEK, NEXT MONTH, NEXT YEAR

Success will come when you take control of your own meals. Decide what you want from the food you eat. If you want mindful, healthy meals, plan a week of varied, nutritious, tasty meals. Once your plan is in place, follow it. Don't be overly ambitious. Choose meals that you'll have time to assemble and write them out on a calendar, preferably one that you already use every day. Make shopping a regular habit. Keep a running list of things you need. Do what you can to make meal planning and preparation easy on yourself. Cook in advance if you have to. Plan where, when, and with whom you'll eat (this is a big one because it makes eating your meal about more than the food).

It's all in the planning

It may seem crazy to break down every detail of planning your meal. You're an adult. You've gotten by so far. But look at the results! Look, we aren't all born knowing how to feed ourselves good food. It's a learned skill, and sometimes it needs to be relearned. If the thought of planning menus for your family strikes terror into your heart, take a deep breath and think again, because it really isn't as tough as it sounds. A good plan means that you know in advance what you're eating. It makes shopping quick and efficient. And, best of all, you're never going to find yourself staring blankly into the refrigerator again saying, "I have absolutely no idea what we're having for dinner tonight — let's order takeout."

During the next month, make sure that you set aside some time each week to plan the menu for the following week. Try to do this at the same time each week and, if possible, immediately follow it up with a trip to the supermarket to purchase what you will need. Keep in mind that you only need to plan four weeks of menus initially — then repeat. This can be the template that you use to get into the rhythm of preparing and eating healthy nutritious meals at home. As you find new and interesting meals, you can bring new favorites into rotation and expand your repertoire to continually mix it up for you and your partner or family.

Dear Peter:

By decluttering and organizing my life, kitchen included, I have been on a much more balanced, healthy diet. I plan my meals in advance and never have I written down "McDonald's" or "chocolate cake" as a meal plan. I try to keep a backup plan in the house for when something unexpected happens — like if the pork chops I intended to cook went bad or if I feel ill. My backup plans might not be the healthiest — fettuccine Alfredo or grilled cheese sandwiches — but they aren't terrible. Being planned and organized in the kitchen and my life really makes a difference in my life for the types and amounts of food I eat. I feel more in control of my life, body, and emotions.

If you don't live alone, be sure to keep in mind the family schedule. Is there a night when someone regularly works late or has sports training until well after the regular mealtime?

Tailor your meals for these occasions so that what you have prepared can easily be served to the latecomers. Variety is also important, as is keeping it real. Don't plan a three-course dinner if you know that it's well beyond what is reasonable to prepare in the time you have. Simple meals can be easy, delicious, and quick to make. Casseroles can be prepared well in advance. Maybe now is the time to pull that slow cooker out of the cupboard where it's been sitting unused for way too long.

In planning menus, focus on balance: lean protein, whole grains, vegetables, and fruits. Plan side dishes that can quickly be prepared by you or a family member right before the meal and served straight to the table. A new dish every few weeks is a good idea — it keeps everyone guessing and lets you try your hand at something new.

Think ahead as you're planning your menus. If you're preparing chicken for one meal, consider cooking some extra for another dish later in the week. Similarly with casseroles, chili, or other meals that will freeze easily — cook twice as much as you need, eat half, and freeze the rest. But make sure you include the leftovers in your upcoming menu; otherwise, you'll just be creating food clutter. And be sure to clearly label what's in that freezer bag and the date you made it. It'll make life a lot easier down the track.

Pick recipes that make sense

Everyone needs inspiration! Maybe you don't think of yourself as a cookbook person, but remember that you have to start somewhere in deciding what meals you would like to prepare and eat at home. Enjoying a variety of foods is really important to help you stay focused so you eat appropriately. When you are the one doing the preparation you know what you are eating, so it's easier to make healthy choices. By using either a good cookbook, or by finding great recipes on the Web, you can take the guesswork out of knowing what you are going to eat.

Expand your horizons by gradually finding simple new recipes that make lean proteins and vegetables as tasty as a Quarter Pounder. Tear recipes out of magazines, find them online, or pick one cookbook you like and try one new recipe every week. Make sure to choose recipes that aren't complex. If the recipe calls for two different cooking methods (for example, steaming then sautéing), you're in for twice the pot washing. Who needs that? Make "low-maintenance" dishes — meals that, once prepared, just go in the oven instead of needing constant attention. Look for cookbooks that have simple menus, with a reasonable number of ingredients that you quickly recognize. Meals that can be prepared in thirty minutes or so make more sense for busy people. Check out Rachael Ray's *30-Minute Meals* cookbooks or similar titles that focus on simplicity, speed, and nutrition. These are a great source of tasty, easy-to-prepare healthy meals that you can enjoy putting together and have a great time eating!

Do you hate dealing with raw meat? Find vegetarian recipes, or do the meat first to get it over with. Better yet, find a dish that needs to marinate and have your partner deal with the meat the night before.

Once the recipes are chosen and the shopping is done, you've saved yourself all that time staring into the refrigerator wondering what you're going to eat. All you need to do is walk in the door and get the pot boiling, the oven preheating, or the microwave zapping. As dinner cooks you can go through the mail, straighten up the kitchen, make a phone call, or catch up with your partner.

Use a sturdy binder, folder, or even an expanding file to store your recipes. You'll easily be able to find them for future reference and over time you'll create a collection of most-favorite dishes.

Avoid convenience foods

Convenience food, usually prepackaged frozen food, promises to make our lives easier. Just stick it in the microwave and ten minutes later — presto! — dinner. It's simple. It saves time. It must be good. Convenience foods may save you time and effort in the short term, but the long-term results are not ideal. Most of these foods are over-processed, which means they lose nutrients. They're often high in sodium, other preservatives, and chemicals. Check the ingredients list: If it doesn't sound like a food, don't eat it.

Shop for meals, not for food

Your days of browsing the grocery aisles are over! Now that you are using your weekly meal calendar to make your shopping list, there should not be much difference between the two. All the shopping list does is break down the meals in to ingredients. If you want to eat snacks, be sure to put them on your meal calendar and on your shopping list. Your list should be so clearly written that a stranger could follow it. If there are certain foods that are on your list week after week, I suggest making them into a master list and photocopying it so you don't have to rewrite the same items every week. Be very careful with your list. Pay attention to how much you need, and if you end up throwing food away, make a mental note to buy less next time. I want you to be thorough. When you get to the checkout, be sure to cling tightly to the shopping cart — it's the best way to avoid any of those chocolate bars that are calling your name just as you get to the register!

FOOD-CLUTTER PRINCIPLE

Figure out what your goal is for your body. If a food doesn't serve that goal, don't eat it.

Stick to the list

The most important rule for shopping is to *only buy what's on your list.* A grocery store is a place of temptation. Food is on display: aisles and aisles of cookies and cakes and brownies and ice cream and potato chips and butterballs and God knows what else. There are so many temptations that if you escape with just a container of ice cream and a bag of chocolate chip cookies, you feel proud of yourself. This is why you have your list. Remember: You are the boss of a world governed by logic, balance, and proportion. You made the list. You didn't put ice cream on the list for a reason. This time you're going to listen to yourself instead of to the marketing ploys of crafty food distributors. Stick to the list. It is you at your strongest.

Stay on the perimeter

The healthiest foods in the grocery store are the ones that are as close as possible to their natural state. Just-picked fruit, just-harvested vegetables and grains, just-slaughtered meat (sorry, had to say it). These foods are generally stocked in a U around the perimeter of the grocery store, so start your shopping there. Fill up your cart with colorful, healthy, fresh-grown foods.

When and where

Make things easier on yourself: Don't shop when you're hungry. You'll be more likely to cheat on your list. Don't shop when you're exhausted or you'll come home with bags of frozen dinners because you can't imagine ever having the energy to cook anything. Remember, you are buying food, not the airbrushed pictures of the food on the boxes in the freezer section, the "serving suggestion" created by food stylists. The more you can make your shopping trips routine, the better. If your shopping trip is part of your routine, built into your schedule, then it's easier for you to build good habits around it. In my own family, we do the grocery shopping on late-afternoon Sundays. The supermarket is quiet, it's the time the store unpacks fresh produce for the week, we aren't hungry, and we're relaxed enough at the end of the weekend to think creatively about the meals we'll eat during the week. It all makes for a more pleasant and efficient shopping excursion. We shop at the same store at the same time every week — trust me, it makes life a lot easier and meal preparation a lot simpler.

When you come home

Unpacking your groceries may seem like a no-brainer, but we often do it in such a rush that we make our lives harder and end up wasting time and food. If you haven't already, scan the refrigerator and throw out any food that's too old, then move food that needs to be used immediately to the front.

As you unpack, put the old foods in front of new ones so you don't have to think about which carton of milk to grab.

When you arrive home with the groceries, you're immediately assaulted with the other demands of home — the ringing phone, e-mails, snail mail, family members wanting your attention. Resist! As you unload the groceries, clean and dry your vegetables and fruits before storing them. You're doing a favor for your later self. Now you can grab a bunch of grapes to nibble without thinking twice.

If you bought high-risk foods — such as snack foods that are okay in small quantities but disastrous if you eat the whole package — then divide it out and store it in proper portions. A much-hungrier you will open this refrigerator later. Do whatever it takes to remind that weaker you to stick to your plan.

Write it out

Now start all over again. Write out your meal plan for the week ahead. Take your appointments for that week into account. If you're going out to dinner one night, plan to eat extra lightly that day. If you plan to make enough for leftovers one night, schedule them in for lunch the next day. Be realistic. You can't easily go from living on takeout to making home-cooked meals every night of the week (or without wanting my head on a platter!), so know yourself. Plan for nights out and mindful indulging. Remember — it's all in the planning!

Did all go according to plan?

After your first week of planning, look back and assess what you wrote in your calendar and your food journal. How did it work out for you? Did you cook all those meals? Did you enjoy them? Did you feel pleased with the meal — how it tasted and how much pleasure you got from it, both while you were eating and afterward? Circle meals that were successful and transfer them to your calendar for next week. Note why certain meals didn't happen as planned or never happened at all. Were you too busy? Too tired? Uninspired? Did you eat better this week than you did the week before? Did you feel better about your eating choices? What can you do better next week? You're not trying to be perfect, you're trying to change. Did you take even the smallest step toward being the ideal you? Take another one next week.

CHECKLIST FOR CHAPTER SIX

- ❑ Take the Are You a Planner? quiz.
- ❑ List what you know about the foods you eat.
- ❑ Create a menu for next week.
- ❑ Get rid of any "Yesterday" foods in your home.
- ❑ Shop with a list.
- ❑ Assess: Did all go according to plan?

Seven:
The Meals You Prepare

What Do You Want From Dinner?
We've talked about the spaces where you store and prepare your food. We've made a plan for what to eat and how to shop for it. Now we're getting to the big moment: the meal itself. What purpose does it serve? How does it contribute to the life you want for yourself? How is it prepared? Where does it take place? Is the space warm, comfortable, and as nourishing as the food on your plate? How about the company and the atmosphere? How do they make you feel? As we explore these questions, keep in mind what you want from your meals. What changes do you need to make to where and how they occur? Remember: Eating out, eating fast food, snacking, and eating takeout make you fat, but preparing healthy, nutritious meals at home will help you lose weight. The only way to motivate yourself to eat at home is to create an experience that

makes you happy.

Ah, your nice, clean, cheerful kitchen. Now it's time to get it messy.

"What's for dinner?" It's the common refrain at the end of the day. But here is the challenge: I want you to ask yourself not "What do I want *for* dinner?" but rather "What do I want *from* dinner?" What do you want *from* the meals you eat? When you finish eating, what is it you want to take *from* the table? What's the purpose of the meals you eat? These are questions we seldom ask ourselves or think about. Sure, we eat to survive, but beyond that, what is it you want *from* the meals you enjoy?

Dear Peter:

My ideal atmosphere would be to eat in a completely separate room from the kitchen that is also away from the rest of the house. I would love it to be a setting that is just purposed for eating, so each dinner feels special. I would have warm colors, interesting pictures on the wall, and lots of candlelight. It would be a time where my husband and I could talk with quieter voices and savor every bite and word together.

Traditionally, meals have been opportunities for people to gather, where stories were told, where the history of a family was passed on from one generation to the next. The dinner table was where children learned about who they were and where they came from, where values were imparted and culture communicated. Gathering around a table was about far more than the food that was consumed. It was about strengthening ties, sharing lives, and bonding through common experiences. It was about learning, sharing, and the experience of the group.

> Dear Peter:
> What is the atmosphere of my ideal meal with loved ones? In my home with a dining area large enough to have about five or six people around. A meal prepared by me in a home that could be described as clean, welcoming, and unburdened by what I see in others as the "need" to have the latest/biggest/best of everything. The atmosphere must be welcoming — a word that keeps coming back.

So what about the dinners you eat? How does dinner fit into the structure of your social life? What is it that you want from your meals? To eat as quickly as possible and then move on to "important" things? To avoid the people you live with? To deprive yourself of what you like to eat because it's "bad" for you? Or is it to end the day with a sense of well-being and accomplishment? To share experiences and grow with the people you care about? To tell jokes and make noise? To talk about successes and aspirations? To eat good food? There are thousands of possible answers. What are yours?

ACTIVITY

Decide what you want from *a meal*

THREE THINGS I WANT *FROM* MY DINNER?

1._____

2._____

3._____

I'm starting with dinner in part because it's often a time when we're tired from a long day. When we don't have dinner planned, we tend to snack all the way up to the moment of decision. And then we tend to fall back on easy solutions like takeout, fast food, or frozen prepackaged convenience meals. Plus, I'm focusing on dinner because, of all your encounters with food throughout the day, the week, the month, and your life, it seems like the one you should make sure to get right. Dinner is a real opportunity for pleasure and I want you to take advantage of it. Think about how life adds up. When you look back on your life, instead of pointing to holidays and vacations as memorable moments, I want you to be able to say, "I always loved dinner at home."

FOOD-CLUTTER PRINCIPLE

Recognize and celebrate every meal you enjoy. It will remind you of the great things a meal provides, beyond just the food.

DON'T JUST EAT — ENJOY!

Be present in the moment. That means being aware of who you are, where you are, who you're with, what you're eating, and how it all fits into the life you want for yourself. Don't count every bite and how many times you chew it. You've been working hard to find meals that satisfy you without packing on pounds. I also want you to be able to step back and make sure you haven't lost your ability to enjoy your meal. I want you to find a calm awareness. We know how to eat — eating is the mechanical action of placing food into your mouth, chewing, and swallowing it. But isn't that exactly what your pet does? If there isn't a significant difference between how your pet eats and how you consume food, then something is seriously wrong.

In this culture, the delivery and consumption of food in a quickly as possible manner has become one measure of a successful meal. What's your reaction if you sit down in a restaurant and a server doesn't come to the table within sixty seconds? Annoyance? Anger? Even outrage? I've seen people completely lose their cool over this. Frankly, it drives me nuts. When you sit down at the table, stop. Take a breath. Appreciate the moment, enjoy the people you're with, then savor your food. The opportunity to talk and laugh and interact with your family and friends is as important as the food itself.

Dear Peter:
    While in France we stayed with families who did not just stuff their houses with clutter like they seem to do in America.

223

They had few pieces of furniture inherited from their families and teacups were hung — not stuffed into a cupboard with four sets of different dishes. They served wonderful food, but they took a long, relaxing time to eat the meals. There was no rushing. I think that is more where the French paradox comes in, rather than the French wine (I don't happen to like wine). After more than a week of cheese and pastries and sauces, etc., I came home at least five pounds lighter.

A lost tradition: giving thanks

I'm not a particularly religious person but the act of saying grace or giving thanks before a meal is an ancient tradition that served an important function. Don't dismiss this idea too quickly if you're not religious as the lesson here has nothing to do with faith. The expression of a common prayer forced everyone at the table to stop, pause, and reflect. It focused everyone's attention on the moment when the whole world is reduced to those who gather around a table to share the fellowship of a meal. At the same time it was a reminder to be thankful for good food, and to think of the often complicated world beyond that table.

I'm not suggesting that we all start saying grace before meals, but it can't hurt to give thanks in some way for what you have. Be mindful of the food you are eating, the company you are sharing, and how each contributes to creating the life you want for yourself. Think of it as a little Thanksgiving every day. Don't just enjoy the food, be aware of it, appreciate the experience.

Slow down

When you finish what's on your plate, don't rush to get seconds. Wait. Take your time. Discuss it with yourself. Do you really need more to sustain your body, or are you stuck in the eating zone? Get up from the table and wash all the dishes. Are you really so hungry that you're willing to start all over and dirty another set of dishes? Wouldn't these leftovers make a great lunch tomorrow? Finally, and this is the hardest part for some of us, don't reward yourself for eating such a wonderfully healthy meal by indulging in ice cream or other desserts. What are those things doing in your house anyway? How do they serve your goals? Get them out of there! You ate your meal. You're done. You're busy — so get back to all those critically important activities that were taking up all your meal preparation time. Go live your ideal life.

THE OTHER MEALS

Breakfast

Granted, it's hard to summon the same level of organization and ritual for meals other than dinner. The point is to get into the habit of deciding what you want an occasion to be, and doing what it takes to make it happen. So if breakfast is the only time your whole family can be together, focus on breakfast. If breakfast in your home is hurried and slapdash, think about whether that is your ideal. What makes it so hectic? Do you need to get up earlier? Do you need to do more preparation the night before? Does every family member eat something different? Is everyone helping out in the morning or are you trying to juggle making breakfast, packing lunches, and corralling unruly children?

For some people, breakfast is a tough meal to get excited about. It's easier to grab something fast — a shot of caffeine and the quick rush of sugar from a muffin or pastry — and hit the ground running. But I want you to think about it this way. Almost everyone likes routine in the morning. What I want you to make sure of is that the morning autopilot you've programmed is a good one. Your day starts when you wake up. When you eat breakfast you set the tone for the day. Make sure you've decided how you want to handle breakfast, and make sure it works for you. You don't want a breakfast doughnut setting your vision for the day.

If you have kids, set a good example for them. Remember all those studies about breakfast being so critical. Yeah, yeah, yeah: breakfast is the most important part of the day. You've heard it a million times. You can mock them all you want, but your body does need to refuel every day, and if you don't like to eat breakfast for yourself, you might want to have another go at it for the sake of your children. When you send your child out the door with a stomach full of good food he can focus better, listen more attentively, learn more quickly, and generally perform much better than the child who skipped breakfast in favor of the vending machine at school. (Same goes for you, by the way — eat a good breakfast and you won't fall prey to those cravings before lunch.)

If a change in how you eat breakfast is in order, sit down and discuss it with the whole family. We're talking about the happiness, success, and growth of the people you love the most here. Show your kids what you believe to be important and model that behavior for them. Commit to it and you'll see instant results.

Lunch and snacks

Lunch and snacks for most of us don't happen at home anymore. If you have trouble planning lunches and snacks in advance, try keeping track of what you eat and what you feed your kids in a small notebook over two weeks' time. When you've finished, look back on the two weeks. Do you like what you see? Is everyone eating healthy foods? Are the foods fresh? Is there variety and flavor? If you see foods you don't like — a pack of chips here, a candy bar there — cross them out and write in healthy substitutions. There! Done! You have your next two weeks of lunches and snacks, ready to go.

Balance your lunches

Write down the lunches you eat most frequently. Which ones are good for you? Which ones are not the healthiest choices you could make? And if you're indulging at lunch, ask yourself, Am I eating too much at lunch because I skimped at breakfast? Remember that eating lunch in front of your computer is basically the same as eating dinner in front of the TV. You are not eating mindfully, so it's easy to lose track of how much you're eating. If you eat while you're reading e-mail or a magazine, you'll end up eating more as you finish.

PREPARING THE MEAL

One way to make sure healthy, delicious food is quickly available when you come home from work or are too tired to cook is to prepare food in advance. Make time on a weekend (or whenever you have time off) to cook a few dishes that will last well through the week. Don't worry about side dishes. Make a stew or a roast chicken. Experiment. Even if you hate to cook, you may find that when you make cooking an activity that you do when you're relaxed, with no pressure, it starts to be more fun. And the more you cook, the more comfortable you'll be. You'll learn how to prepare certain favorite dishes that keep well over the work week. You'll be able to invite a friend over on the spur of the moment, knowing that you have an easy meal you can reheat. Always make sure you put a reasonably-sized portion on your plate and don't go back for more. It's no good if you eat a whole week's worth of food at one meal. Imagine how great it will be to pull out a dinner you made, knowing the healthy ingredients that went into it.

Plan foods to cook in advance

Foods that I could make and freeze for future use:

- _____
- _____
- _____
- _____
- _____
- _____

Cooking in the moment

Of all the rooms in your home, the kitchen is the one where you absolutely must finish what you start. If you dirty a dish, put it in the dishwasher, not on the counter or sink. If you empty something, fill it. If you take something out, put it back. Clean and clear as you go so that work surfaces are never cluttered and the kitchen is a place you want to be, before, during, and after you cook.

The first step to cooking well is to start in a clear and clean space. Then — and this is critical — put on music that you enjoy. Choose music that gives you energy and makes you happy. Some people like to watch TV while they cook, but as far as I'm concerned, watching TV says that you're bored and need to multitask, and it's easy to get distracted from the task at hand. I want you to get *into* cooking. I want you to make it fun or meditative, a time of day you look forward to because you don't have to think too hard. You're active, engaged, working with fresh, healthy ingredients, and creating delicious meals, so choose music that puts you in the mood and helps you focus on the task at hand.

Now pull out the recipes and ingredients you plan to use for the meal. These are the recipes you chose when you made your shopping list. Unless it's a special occasion, keep everything simple. Nobody can cook a gourmet meal every single night. Besides, simple foods made from fresh ingredients are healthy and taste good. In my family we go by the theory that the less you mess with fresh ingredients, the better the meal will be. If the recipes you chose work, mark the page or add the recipe to next week's meal plan. If you cook a favorite meal a few times, you'll get used to making it and remember it as an option in the future. Just don't overdo it or you'll never want to taste that delicious pesto chicken again.

Enlist help if it's available. Ask the kids to set the table or measure out ingredients. Cooking is full of mini-math lessons for schoolkids. Make the meal into family to-gether time. If you make an elaborate main dish, be sure to keep your side dishes easy. Steam vegetables and rice, or make a quick salad of mostly greens.

Remember — get into the routine of clean-ing the kitchen as you go, using the time when food is cooking to straighten up and do any dishes you've generated. By the time dinner is ready, the only things you'll have left to clean are a couple pots or serving dishes, and the dishes you use to eat.

Don't invest too much in the product. Focus on the process instead. Trying new recipes is always an experiment, and if it doesn't turn out as good as it sounded, well, you've learned a little something. If not everyone likes what you made, don't let it get to you. Your time wasn't wasted. Discovering new foods is important.

The hamburger experience is so narrow. It narrows your thinking in all ways. It's not just about the food. It's about everything.
Alice Waters, *The Delicious Revolution*

FAST FOOD

Alice Waters is the widely respected chef of the restaurant Chez Panisse in Berkeley, California. She is known for using only high-quality, in-season foods that are organically grown in ecologically sound ways. The food at her restaurant comes mostly from local farmers. All this is a reflection of her outlook on life. This chef speaks of food and celebration and the meal as some people speak about a lover. When I first heard Alice Waters talk about "the hamburger experience," I stopped dead in my tracks: What we eat is a reflection of our experience of the world. When we eat the same thing day after day, our senses become dulled and our outlook is severely restricted. If you are what you eat, consider what effect a diet composed mainly of hamburgers from a fast-food restaurant can have on you. The artificial sweeteners, chemical additives, meat mixed from hundreds of force-fed animals all serve the profit of big business. Can this diet be good for you? Moreover, eating fake food in a generic environment must affect your vision for yourself. What kind of person do you want to be?

Dear Peter:

It is my opinion that my family and I eat out either at restaurants or zip through the drive-through for a meal far more than I think we should, for no other reason than the clutter in our kitchen/cooking area makes it tough (if not impossible — some days are like that, too) to productively and comfortably get a meal together and on the table for all of us to enjoy together (there are four of us: mom, dad, two daughters, and our third baby is on the way in December!).

When it comes to fast food, you can't win. You can argue or rationalize, but the bottom line is that fast food simply is not good for you. It's like filling your home with cheap, poor quality, spontaneous purchases that clutter your space and overwhelm you. Fast food, cheap clutter — they're not so different. Sure, all the fast-food restaurants are introducing healthy options, and if that works for you, great. But the best-tasting options in fast-food restaurants are the ones that are bad for you. Like it or not, there is no simple way to put this. With fast food, the guidelines are simple and brutal:

No supersizing/combos
No sauce
No cheese
No bacon
No dressing
Nothing fried
No dessert

You can count calories, order chicken salads, get diet soda, but it's all a waste of time. Your best bet is to just stay away. Period.

Soda

Like fast food, soda also has to go. Soda has become a staple of the American diet, each of us drinking an average of two and a half cans every day. In regular soda that's seventy-one pounds of pure sugar every year from soda alone! Does that sound healthy to you? Put a little differently, when the calories from just two cans of soda a day are added to your normal diet, you'll find yourself adding close to thirty-five pounds of extra weight in a year. It also appears that drinking as little as one can of soda a day — diet or regular — can greatly increase your risk for heart disease and diabetes. The phosphoric acid in soda also appears to weaken bones by depleting calcium from your system. Whether it's the extra weight or the tooth decay, the high levels of caffeine, or the risk of weakened bones, the message is clear. As tough as it sounds, if you're serious about moving toward a healthier life, the soda has to go.

Takeout

Banish takeout. What's so bad about takeout, you ask? "I order from pretty healthy places," you insist. But here's what I'm trying to tell you: Don't make this about the food. It's about what the decision to eat takeout says about the life you are choosing to live.

Takeout is food prepared by others, without your involvement, with ingredients you have no control over, in portions that are too big for one meal. It's about mass production. Think of it as junk mail. It comes into your house pretending to offer you something you want, but if you don't stop it at the door, it just keeps coming. It's nothing like real correspondence — like bills and personal letters — which you may not look forward to but at least know are important communications. You have no idea whether junk mail contains stuff you want or don't want (I can tell you — you don't want it), but it just keeps coming until it takes over your home. Same goes with take-out food. Yes, it only takes a phone call from you to invite it into your home, but is it something you want or need? Much of the food is so processed it's more "food substitute" than real food. Is this the life you really want to live? A life to which you are not connected and over which you have little control? Is this the life you imagined for yourself?

It's a free country. You decide what food to put into your body. But with the food comes consequences. Consistently choosing to eat fast food or takeout rather than cooking for yourself says a great deal:

- I didn't take the time to plan this meal.
- I'm making a choice to do what is easiest, not what is best for me.
- I'm eating food that someone else made. I have no idea what went into it or whether it's good for me and I don't care.
- Mealtime isn't important to me. I just want to eat. I'd rather not think about what we're having, and I'm probably not thinking about whether the time is spent pleasurably.

You're trying to lose weight. You've chosen meals that are good for you and serve your goals. You have a plan. If you want to see results you need to stick to the plan. Talk to me about takeout if you're happy with your life. Talk to me about fast food and takeout after you've lost all the weight you want to lose. Until then, trust me, it's a slippery slope paved in fat and sodium.

THE COMPANY YOU KEEP

Eating alone

When we eat alone we tend to let all our ideas about how a meal should taste, what it should consist of, how it should be served, and what the experience as a whole should be go out the window. Nobody's watching, so it's easy to revert to eating an entire pint of ice cream and calling it dinner, or to scarfing down an enormous burrito on the go. Yes, it's harder to justify going to the effort to prepare a healthy meal for you and only you. But this is about you! You're the one who's trying to change. Going it solo is a great opportunity to make the meal exactly what you want it to be.

If and when you're eating alone, I want you to remind yourself of the life you want to live. Are you that nonthinking person downing a greasy fast-food cheeseburger, or are you willing to take the extra five minutes to prepare a salad that will give you the energy you need for the rest of the day and will be part of a wholesome diet that over the years adds up to better health and happiness? Make eating alone a ritual you enjoy. Relish the solitude. Put on music. As you get your healthy, visually appealing meal together, remind yourself that when you are done eating you won't have to face any feelings of guilt. You can be proud. You can walk around for the rest of the day feeling energized (and telling yourself that you feel thinner already). You can relax after dinner without thinking about all the day's extra calories that you should be burning off.

Most people go solo for lunch. Sure, you might have company — a lunch date or a meal in the cafeteria with coworkers. But many of us eat at our desks. Remember: It's up to you and you alone to make choices about how and where you spend that time, and what you put in your mouth. Consider the siestas that are common in tropical cultures all over the world. Though we all think of a siesta as a nap, the original meaning was a midday break, an opportunity to spend time with family and friends. In our culture, lunch is our only opportunity to refuel and reenergize for the day. You think this is best achieved by wolfing down some fast food from a carton in front of your computer or eating your children's leftovers while you clean up? Not likely. You need a break. A true break. You deserve one. It will improve your performance for the rest of the day. Don't let lunch happen to you; plan it. Put it on your calendar at work. Call it a doctor's appointment if you must. Everyone will think you're seeing a therapist, and you know what? The results might be just as good and a whole lot cheaper. If you're the parent of small children, or your work is otherwise ceaseless and uncompromising, you must be even more organized. It's tough to put together a meal when you're tending kids, so you need to have a healthy meal all ready and waiting for you. Try making it the night before. It's good practice for packing school lunches anyway.

Taking charge of the meals that you eat when you're alone may be the hardest thing I'm asking you to do. When we are alone, our greatest fears and anxieties tend to surface. To push them away, we clutter our time. We minimize alone time or camouflage it in distractions or sit in front of the TV for hours with our minds in stand-by mode. To really claim that mealtime and make it a solitary pleasure is a tough challenge. To do it regularly, to make it part of the way you live your life, is a commitment. It's a commitment to bringing peace and order to your day. It's a commitment to valuing yourself and savoring the life you have chosen. It's a commitment to your best life.

If you are not alone by choice, you may be resistant to enjoying your time alone because it's not what you want. I understand that, but by now don't we all know that loneliness fades if you embrace your life? Search for a real state of mind where you enjoy your own company first. If you want to meet a partner, you up your chances by finding peace and making a life for yourself that someone else would be able to join with pleasure.

Eating with a partner

Dear Peter:
My husband and I have no children yet, so mealtime is usually quiet. I do all the cooking myself and I try to have it ready so when my husband gets home from work all we have to do is sit down and dig in. We are very involved with our church, and are out several times a week. Since we are on a schedule, we usually don't have a long time to eat, but we try to make the minutes count. While we're eating it's all about enjoying the good food and each

other. We talk about our day and sometimes silly stuff. Even if we have just
twenty minutes, we're always refreshed
and happy afterward.

If you are building a life with a partner, your
shared goals and direction have to be something you work on. Your food choices should
also be part of this discussion. Decide with
your partner which of your meals it makes
sense to eat together. Do you divvy up tasks,
like shopping, prepping, cooking, and cleaning? Are you both happy with the division of
responsibilities? Are you both happy with the
meals that result from your efforts? If not,
one way to get on the same page is to literally get on the same page. Flip through
cookbooks together. Sometimes if a person
is resistant to healthy food choices, it's because they assume it means plain chicken
breast with steamed vegetables night after
night. Start by finding a few meals that
sound good to both of you. Plan a week
around them. Ask friends and family for favorite healthy recipes. Go to a gourmet
health store to remind yourself that with the
right recipe a salmon filet or skinless chicken
breast can be miraculously transformed.

Discuss with your partner/family what you all want *from* your meals

What meals do we share?

How/when do we decide what to eat?

Who does the shopping? Prepping? Cooking? Cleaning?

Do we both/all like the division of responsibilities?

Do we like the food we eat?

Where do we eat? Is it pleasant?

What do we do while eating? Talk? Watch TV?

Do we enjoy the meals we have together?

What would you change about the meals we share?

What do you want from dinner?

Eating with family

When you and your partner were alone, you could chat while making dinner. You probably had whole weekends to enjoy without significant responsibilities. When kids come along, it becomes much harder to gather the whole family in one place. Everyone has different schedules, different commitments, and different tastes. You have to work hard to make meals a central event, a place where familial bonds are established and secured.

We keep returning to the question that drives my whole approach: What is the life you want? What life does your family want? Imagine how you would like a meal with your family to look and feel. Is it leisurely and calm, with civilized conversation and light storytelling? Is it exuberant and messy, with people talking on top of each other, jokes being told, drinks being spilled, and a dog vacuuming up underfoot? Or is your family a line of people sitting silently on the couch, staring vacantly at some violent drama or not-so-funny sitcom rerun as they grab slices of pizza? TV will make them fat. Save them now!

Dear Peter:

I have noticed in the past year that our family of four is busier than ever, and we are no longer eating together at the table. Mainly this is because we would starve before we cleared the clutter off the dining room table and because we have run out of space to move the junk to. So we eat in front of the TV in the living room. I think we

---

eat more and we snack more, partly because we are out of the routine of eating together as a family. It's hard to make sure everyone eats their salad and vegetables when they have to get their own food right off the stove and they can pick and choose what they want. And the more we eat like this, the more I feel guilty and responsible for my husband's weight gain (about twenty pounds). If he had a heart attack now I would never forgive myself.

My dream is to have my husband come home from working his twelve-to-fourteen-hour day and be happy to see his home and dinner on the table. If I was more in control I could kiss him hello with cheerfulness and help him to de-stress from his day.

One of the biggest single reasons I see for the spread of clutter through homes is the total absence of any sense of routine in the family's life. Kids have activities that change every night and occupy the hours between school and bedtime. Sometimes just getting them fed, even if it's with fast food on the way home from sports practice, seems like an achievement. But ask yourself why you let that happen: Are you treating their bodies with respect? Are they? The behavior you get from your children is the behavior you model yourself. Children grow to respect and value what their parents respect and value. It's a question I frequently ask parents: "If you don't teach your children about the place of food in their lives, the importance of respectful conversation, and the value of shared experiences, who will?"

I was recently invited to dinner by Adam and Joanne, a couple I know, at a great Italian restaurant that we all enjoy. When I arrived I was surprised to discover that they had also brought their two sons — ages nine and eleven. I had assumed it was an adults-only affair. From the moment we sat down, however, I was fascinated by the attitude and behavior of the two boys. Here were two young men — not yet teenagers — who knew exactly how to conduct themselves at a meal table. At first they were shy, but once I started asking them about school, favorite sports, and current computer games, they really warmed up. Even when they got excited or wanted to press a point, they were careful not to interrupt each other or the rest of us at the table. Each of them ordered from the menu, asked to have their glasses refilled when necessary, and knew how to use a knife and fork correctly.

When I commented on the boys' behavior to their parents, they explained that they had agreed very early on to make the meal table a central part of their family life. Mealtime became family time. Adam and Joanne take the boys to dinner with them as frequently as they can, even though this is at times unpopular with their adult friends. They encourage the boys to try different foods and both explain and model the behavior they expect from them in a restaurant. It doesn't always work out the way they'd like — kids are kids and even the best-laid plans can go wrong. But the habits the boys are developing now will be with them for the rest of their lives.

The dinner table is where the tone for your family is set. Plan the meal. Involve the family. Be mindful of what you eat. Enjoy one another. Health, respect, open lines of communication — the benefits are enormous.

Filter the voices

Who are the people closest to you? How do they play into the choices you make? Do you and your husband like to curl up on the couch in front of the TV with heaping plates of takeout? Does your mother criticize your weight every time she sees you? Does your wife pinch your love handles and say, "I must really love you a *lot.*" Does your spouse love to cook delicious food that's contributing five pounds a year to your waistline? Do you and your best friend always go out for ice cream? Amazingly, recent research has found that having friends who are obese can nearly triple your own chances of becoming fat. Fat isn't contagious, but clearly social and family networks have a strong influence on your weight.

These are the people who love us most. Love is care, but it can also be indulgence. Indulgence doesn't always breed the healthiest choices. Here is the first, and possibly the hardest, choice you're going to have to make: You need to be sure that your relationships serve your new goals. If they don't, it's time to do some adjusting.

Dear Peter:

To stick to my low-calorie diet I have to grit my teeth when out with my husband. He often stops for french fries, pizza, and other snacks, and always offers some to me. He isn't trying to be mean, because in his family, food was a treat. In my family, food was food.

Remember: Your body is *your* responsibility. Your voice should be the most powerful one in your head. Change comes from within you. Take a close look at the role your relationships play in your food decisions. Do the people in your life prod you to eat more, or poorly? Does their criticism provoke you? Can they support you as you try to make changes?

Dear Peter:

My second husband does not help the matter [of my weight difficulties]. He is also overweight. He loves to cook and has a lot of those quirky hang-ups — you must try everything, you must clean your plate, you must have seconds or he is insulted. He cannot cook for two. Rather, he literally cooks army-size amounts. We end up with leftovers that spoil.

Decide what you want from your friends and family. Do you need some space from a person to make decisions independently? If you eat as a family, can you find common ground? What compromises need to be made?

Take a moment and think about the things

you might want to change about your family's meal schedule, eating style, or food preparation routine. Specific examples will make talking with your family about change a lot easier. Fill out this chart the best you can.

WHAT I'D LIKE TO CHANGE ABOUT MEALS IN MY HOME

- _____
- _____
- _____
- _____

If you're the primary cook, ask your family if they'd be willing to help you find new foods that are healthier but still satisfying. If you're lucky enough to have someone else who does most of the cooking, you need to have a serious conversation about how to make changes without insulting the chef! Do you need to get more involved in the shopping and food preparation? Would your ice-cream-loving best friend be willing to start another tradition with you — like going for a walk? Enjoy your life. Enjoy your food and take time to congratulate yourself for each healthy meal. Changes are ahead. They'll be easier to make if you're not alone in the wilderness.

WHERE YOU EAT

The table

The place where you eat says a lot about what you want from the meal. Do you stand over the kitchen sink, madly wolfing down a hastily made sandwich? Do you eat at a neatly set table in your kitchen or dining room? Do you eat in front of the TV? Kath and Jim's seven children are grown and have dispersed. Some have started their own families. When they convene for Christmas, it's a huge affair that involves everyone from the grandparents to the smallest child. While the meal is the culmination of the day, it's the preparation that is an amazing thing to watch. It has become a ritual where everyone arrives about three hours before the main meal and congregates in the kitchen. Rather than the traditional meal of turkey and ham, roasted vegetables, and pies, together the family prepares a meal of fresh seafood and maybe eight or ten different salads. Everyone stands around catching up, having a few drinks, and preparing a different part of the meal. The celebration is as much in the preparation as in the eating. The whole process is a reflection of the love and energy and values of the family. Once the preparation is complete, everyone moves to the table where the food, along with the conversation, bad jokes, and family folklore is shared. It can be a real madhouse, but making the meal generates the joy of the whole event. This celebration has worked for as long as Kath can remember. It's about so much more than what you eat — it's about what nourishes your family.

Special occasions like Christmas or Hanukkah or Thanksgiving are easy to look at in terms of what they mean to us. I want you to take that way of thinking and apply it to what is normal in your home. If you hurry through meals, what are you saying is more important than nourishing yourself? What does the table where you eat look like? Is it clean and clear of clutter? I keep talking about the vision you have for the life you want. The vision has to find real expression, not only in what you have in your home, but also in what you value in your home. Get rid of the clutter that interferes with that vision.

A cluttered table makes you fat. How? Think about what a cluttered table means about your state of mind. You're too busy to create a nice space for your meal. You're too disorganized to put stuff in its proper place.

You don't respect yourself enough to leave room for something you do for nourishment and pleasure every day of your life. And maybe it says other things about you that only you can figure out. I remember one family that I worked with whose nine-year-old daughter and her younger sister had never seen the surface of the dining room table because of the magazines, bills, old mail, and paper clutter that covered it. The parents complained bitterly about their children's eating habits, but thought nothing of eating dinner every night balancing their plates on their knees in front of the TV.

Perhaps the most startling part of working with this family was the reaction of the girls when the clutter was cleared and for the first time they were able to sit at the dining room table for a meal. The older girl actually burst into tears. She said she had never imagined that they could be a family who sat together for a meal and talked about "nothing special, just anything." Have respect for where you eat. It's not just about the food — it's about the life you live and the life you choose to create.

The place where you eat should be special. If you don't honor and respect this important place and the unique and shared moments with your family, what does that say about what you think is important and valuable? If you can't be bothered to preserve a good table for your household, then it's very unlikely that you will bother to take good care of your body.

TV makes you fat

I've made a career out of TV. In fact, I love working on TV and love watching it. But here's the thing about TV: Great as it might be, it's a one-way invention. Try talking back to the set sometime and see how far you get! TV is intended to push information and entertainment at you. All you have to do is sit and absorb. And one more thing: TV doesn't like competition. You know this is true: When you turn on the TV, all communication ceases. It doesn't matter with whom you're eating or what you are eating; if the TV is on, all your attention is focused on the screen. And when I say all your attention, I mean all of it. Even if you're watching as a group, TV isolates each individual and demands your full attention. You can't practice mindful eating if you're a zombie. Not only do you eat quickly and fail to taste your food, much less enjoy it, but you don't notice when you're full. Whatever's in front of you might as well be popcorn at the movies — you just keep shoving it into your mouth until there is no more.

> Dear Peter:
>
> If there is no room on the dining table (covered with clutter!) to set out a proper meal and eat around the table together, where would one eat? In front of the TV most likely, where one would not pay attention at all to what or how much one would be eating. At the dining table, much of the dining experience is again slowed down with conversations. Eating itself is much more mindful.

I told you to give up TV for a month, and I meant it. No TV. Fill that extra time by actively improving your life: clean house, organize finances, spend time with people you care about. Eating in front of the TV is tough to quit. You enjoy it. I get it. But you need to keep in mind your priorities. I'm telling you that if you don't eat in front of the TV, you won't eat as much. It's math. If you eat less, you'll see a change in your body. Isn't that why you're here?

Final Tips

Mom was right

I told you I wasn't going to burden you with fad diet tricks, but there are a few bits of wisdom I want you to consider. It's easy to believe that the knowledge we have is far superior to that of our parents or grandparents. It's true that the kind of food we eat has changed in the last few generations; my experience, however, is that old wisdom is usually good wisdom, particularly when it comes to eating. Your mother and/or grandmother may have recited some of these famous lines:

Chew your food

It takes about twenty minutes for your stomach to let your brain know that it's had enough food. If you're wolfing down your food, however, that twenty-minute delay can mean another twenty minutes of frenzied overeating. Taking it slowly helps you enjoy the food more and avoid that bloated stomach feeling most of us know far too well.

Eat your vegetables

In my family, it was usually "Eat your broccoli." As kids we were encouraged to eat different types of food, and my mother always made sure that right alongside those bright green peas (or broccoli) there were other vegetables of different colors. It was only much later in life that I discovered that the different colors of fruit and vegetables are

Nature's way of letting us know what nutrients are present. Update "eat your peas" for your family and instead say "eat your colors." Maybe, if you're lucky, they'll listen.

Get a good night's sleep

There is a strong relationship between how much you sleep and how much you weigh. Getting a good night's sleep enables your body to get the rest it needs and gives your system a chance to process the food you eat. When you don't get enough sleep your body needs to produce much more insulin to process your food. High insulin levels cause weight gain. It's a vicious cycle, and it becomes almost impossible to maintain a healthy weight. Your mother may not have been thinking about the insulin — she probably just thought you were a grouch in the morning — but she had the right idea.

Don't fill up on bread

Did your grandmother tell you that too much bread before the meal would "ruin your dinner"? Well, there appears to be a weird connection between eating white bread and being overweight. There are plenty of theories about why this is so — we know it has plenty of calories and little nutritional benefit — but everyone seems to agree that it has something to do with fiber in your diet and the lack of fiber in over-processed grains. Whatever the reason, I think we should just chalk it up to something Grandma knew that we don't!

Don't talk with your mouth full!

Eating meals at a reasonable pace and sharing details of your day go hand in hand. When your mother said to keep your mouth shut when chewing, she wasn't just wary of getting sprayed with half-chewed food. Maybe she had Miss Manners in mind, but she also knew that slowing down and taking time with your meal meant enjoying one another's company, respecting what everyone had to say, and simply creating an environment that wasn't totally chaotic.

Your eyes are bigger than your belly

We tend to put more food on our plates than our bodies need and our stomachs can comfortably hold. Did you know that portions in most restaurants are two to three times larger than they were twenty years ago? Dinner plates in these places are practically the size of a surfboard and laden with enough food for two or three people and, unfortunately, research shows that if it's on the plate, we are more than likely to eat it.

Before you take the first bite of any meal, check out how much is on the plate. Do you need that much food?

What did your mother say to you? An apple a day keeps the doctor away? No dessert until you've finished your meal? Start your day with a good breakfast? You can start listening now. Your mom doesn't have to know.

CHECKLIST FOR CHAPTER SEVEN

- ❑ Decide what you want *from* a meal.
- ❑ List the changes you'd like to make with mealtimes in your home.
- ❑ Discuss with your partner/family what you all want *from* your meals.
- ❑ Plan foods to cook in advance.
- ❑ Balance your lunches.
- ❑ Banish takeout.
- ❑ Listen to your mother.

EIGHT: THE LIFE YOU LIVE

EVERYTHING IS CONNECTED

A compartmentalized life doesn't work for most of us. Home, family, love, work, food, activity, hobbies, rest — if one element is out of whack, everything suffers. Your life should be balanced. It should be a productive life, a social life, a spiritual life, a life where you give and receive love. As I hope I've made clear, I believe that home is the best place to start to make changes that reverberate across all parts of a balanced life. I want you to look at all aspects of your life. But since you're here to lose weight, I want you to look particularly at the physical aspects of your life to see if your body is getting the attention it deserves.

Dear Peter:
   I know the clutter problem has gotten much worse in the last year — and as I

write this, I realize that during that same time period my hate for my job has drastically increased. My cluttering is also a problem at work. I have stuff piled everywhere.

You can't separate the physical, emotional, and spiritual parts of you and compartmentalize them. If one part is affected, they all are. If I get myself disciplined in one area (exercise, eating, etc.), the other areas improve. If I slack off in one area, I slack off everywhere.

An active life

Taking control of your life requires energy. Where does that energy come from? That's right, food. But it also comes from leading an active life. Do you ever have a day when you're busy, busy, busy, but you accomplish many small tasks? You drop off the dry cleaning, go to work, pay bills, help a friend, call your mother to say happy birthday, pick up the car from the shop, come home to cook dinner, sort through the mail, clean up the kitchen, clip your nails, and . . . whew! You're done. If you're running in circles, a day like that is the last straw. But if you're ahead of the game, being efficient and productive is invigorating, isn't it? Nothing cleans out mental clutter better than endorphins. So get moving! Tend to unfinished projects around your house, do some gardening, clean out a closet, wash the car or the dog. Instead of snacking for ten minutes, get the ironing done. You'll be amazed at how much joy and energy you'll discover in accomplishing small tasks.

But whatever you do, don't go shopping. The last thing you need is more clutter.

EXERCISE FOR THE LIFE YOU WANT

Each of us knows that healthier food choices are only part of the picture. We tend to spend so much of our time sitting on our butts that it's no surprise the fat accumulates there. That said, however, you don't have to make huge changes to see a difference. Just like with food, you know what needs to be done here! Walk the stairs instead of taking the elevator. Park a little farther away from the entrance to the mall. Mow the lawn instead of hiring a gardener. Even a ten-minute walk every day can make a significant difference in how you look and feel. To start, identify what small changes you can make in your daily life to increase your physical activity. The benefits are enormous.

Dear Peter:

When I am focused on dieting and working out, the clutter in my house starts to get smaller. Things start to get more organized when I'm taking better care of myself.

Start with some exercise that works for you. It's easy to say "whatever works for you," but I really mean it. You'll get bored with or resist exercise that doesn't fit into what you can afford, how old you are, your body, and your preferences. Options vary depending on where you live. But one thing is true for everyone: You can't lose weight without exercise. Exercise burns fat. But that's not all. As you develop muscle, your metabolism increases, and you burn more fat all day long. There's no magic diet pill that will make you thin, but building your muscles in conjunction with a sound diet is the closest you can get to one. No matter how old you are or what shape you're in, you should include cardiovascular activity and weight-bearing exercise into your life. If you are a passive participant in your life, you can count on stuff (weight and clutter) to pile up around you. Take control. Live your life as an active participant. Fill in the chart below with positive things you know you can do *and* stick to.

ACTIVITY	
Increasing Your Physical Activity	
THINGS I DO NOW	**WHAT I CAN DO TO BE MORE PHYSICALLY ACTIVE**
Watch TV for three hours every night	Take a fifteen-minute walk after dinner
Drive the kids to school	Leave ten minutes earlier and walk the kids to school

Live your life

Exercise doesn't have to be a rigorous program where you alternate sprints around a track with push-ups. If you've always hated exercise, you need to reframe the way you think about it. Exercise is just activity. It's moving your body through space. It's having fun and enjoying yourself. If you don't overdo it or spend ten hours a day on a treadmill facing a blank wall, it can be quite enjoyable. Look for fun social ways to be active. Take dance lessons. Try ice-skating. Plan a picnic. If someone invites you on a hike, don't turn them down. Remember, "hike" is just a sporty word for "walk." You can do it. If a group is playing softball, which you hate, go anyway. You don't have to play. Just enjoy being outside. Offer to help carry gear. Walk around the park or field where the game is taking place. Move. See how it feels.

In the life you want, how active do you imagine yourself being? What can you achieve physically? What activities do you enjoy? This vision should be your goal. Maybe you want to spend every Sunday walking around a lake, then picnicking with friends. Maybe you always enjoyed swimming as a kid but have never bothered to look for a pool nearby. Maybe you should take that salsa class you've always thought about. Meet with friends. Make it so much fun you forget it's supposed to be good for you.

Step it up

Here's where I want you to start. It's easy. Whatever you're currently doing, I want you to increase it. If you're inactive, start small.

Walk. If you walk, add weights or jog. If you already exercise, make sure you vary your routine. If you bike, join a gym or start taking longer rides with a friend. If you go to the gym, try a new sport or test out a different class. If you're shy in public, experiment with exercise videos in the comfort of your home. Some of them are terrible and boring, but if you search around and ask friends you can find a few that suit your ability and personality. Put a few into rotation or before long you'll find yourself holding conversations with the video instructor — though that might also be a sign you're ready to take your activity out of the house and into a more social arena.

Time-savers

If time is at a premium, pop in that work-out video while the dinner is in the oven and don't let anyone tease you; get them to exercise with you instead. Whatever works for you is what works. If you can't block out big enough chunks of time to exercise, you can still work it into your lifestyle. Take the dog for a run instead of a walk. If you have a child, find a group of local moms who work out with strollers. If you can't find one, start one. Park farther from work or cut your commute short and walk a mile every morning. Do leg lifts while you watch TV (and now, admit it, you could be at the gym watching TV). Steal your kids' Wii game console — a great new fat burner that is even finding its way into assisted-living facilities where older people are using it to simulate bowling, tennis, and even baseball. If my eighty-four-year-old mother can get into it, so can you!

NINE:
THE CHALLENGES YOU FACE

We talked about the internal, emotional triggers that cause us to eat foods that are bad for us. Now let's talk about external temptations. What are the everyday situations that make it hard to stick to your plan? In this chapter, we're going to identify your high-risk situations for unhealthy food and talk about how to use organization to avoid or change them forever.

FOOD-CLUTTER PRINCIPLE

The fat didn't appear overnight and won't disappear overnight.

MINDFUL INDULGENCE

I've said it a thousand times: Your home should reflect the person you want to be. If you want to make a change, you have to start with your home. But nobody should be a shut-in. Life is meant to be lived. What's the point of having a beautiful and organized home, a perfect diet, and a perfect body if you don't take part in the art, culture, beauty, activity, and people of this world? You may find that eating at home helps you break bad habits and establish routines, but eventually you're going to have to venture out of your safe haven and into the real world, and the real world complicates everything. Let's talk about external triggers: how to deal with eating out, how to have as much fun as you ever did without compromising your health, and how to plan for the unexpected.

Dear Peter:

I also can say that I DO eat differently when out of the house. My best friend loves to go for ice cream or for dinner out, and I never say no, don't know how. I feel as though sometimes I just don't care.

When you go out to eat, be aware. Remember who you are and who you want to be. If you're happier, you'll lose weight. Be happy. Enjoy the night. Don't special order dry salmon and salad with the dressing on the side. The point isn't to be dessert-free. The point is to gravitate to a weight you enjoy by living a full, balanced life. Weight change is a slow and gradual thing. If you're hoping to change your eating habits for a week or three, then go back to the old ways, take my advice: Don't even start. You're not serious.

For right now, what matters is to get to a place where you consciously think about your ideal self. Where does dessert fit in? It may just be one piece of cake on a plate, but how does that fit with what you know you want and deserve? Each decision is part of the broader choice you are making. Use this quiz to evaluate where you fall on the self-control scale.

QUIZ

Know Your Weaknesses

If the waiter puts a basket of bread on the table, do you
- a) immediately help yourself and eat until the next course comes?
- b) take one piece, then stop?
- c) have none?
- d) ask the waiter to remove the bread?

When it comes to drinking with dinner, do you
- a) sometimes have a cocktail, then share a bottle of wine with your companion(s)?
- b) usually have one glass of wine, beer, or a soda?
- c) stick to water?
- d) drink a diet soda?

At a cocktail or work party, when you see a server with hors d'oeuvres, do you
- a) chase them — who are you to turn down free food?
- b) wait for your favorite to come by?
- c) say no — you'll wait for dinner?
- d) hunt down the inevitable table of crudités and fill up on plain celery sticks?

When you choose from a menu, do you
- a) order the yummiest, most inspiring entrée available — isn't that the point of eating at a good restaurant?
- b) pick an appetizer you love, and a main course that you know is pretty good for you?

    c) choose a salad and a colorful, lean entrée?

    d) special order everything — dressing and sauces on the side?

By the time the busboy takes away your plate

    a) it's empty — you're a member of the clean plate club.

    b) it's sometimes empty, sometimes you take home leftovers, depends on how hungry you are.

    c) it's always got a little something left over — you try to leave enough for tomorrow's lunch.

    d) it's been divided down the center and exactly 50 percent of the food you were served remains exactly where it was.

When it comes to fast food

    a) you eat it, you love it, you can't live without it.

    b) you don't eat it constantly, but when it's the only option you have to admit it's pretty good.

    c) you avoid it, but have found some

healthy options at the places where you do go.

d) you can't believe people put that garbage in their bodies.

At the end of the meal

a) you always order dessert. It's a special occasion!

b) you like to share a yummy dessert.

c) you don't order dessert, but if others do you'll have a bite.

d) you sip tea, no sugar, and watch others pig out.

Score yourself

If your answers were mostly As:

You like to live life to the fullest. Going to a restaurant is a fun, festive occasion and you want to make the most of it. I applaud that attitude, and you sound like exactly the sort of dinner companion I'd enjoy. But — and you knew there was a but coming — it's very possible that being overweight inhibits your ability to live life to the fullest. You're in a quandary. At the same time that you're enjoying life, you're taking away from your life. You can't have your cake and eat it, too.

You need to take the same pleasure in a night out without compromising your health. Sure, eating your favorite foods, drinking freely, and eating whatever you want whenever you want gives you a sense of freedom, of excess, of celebration. But these feelings don't come from what you put into your body. They don't come from whatever is on the waiter's tray. They come from you. *You* bring them to the table.

There is a continuum here. There's no need to drastically change everything you do when you eat out. Look at the B answers to the quiz. These are slightly healthier choices. Use them as a guide to start improving the quality and reducing the quantity of what you consume when you eat out. Be mindful of what you bring to the table. You may be surprised to find that what you eat isn't nearly as important as who you're with and how much fun you have together.

If your answers were mostly Bs:

You know what? You're a pretty reasonable person. You don't indulge for the sake of indulging. You don't throw caution to the wind when you eat out, but you're still tempted by a cheesy pasta or a chocolate dessert every now and then. Who can blame you?

The way you eat works for lots of people.

It works for young people whose metabolisms haven't started to creep, and it works for that jerk — I mean friend — of yours who never seems to gain weight no matter what he eats.

I have no problem with the way you eat and the choices you make, except that they're not working for you. Maybe they did once, but not anymore. The point is no matter how reasonable your behavior is, you're not happy with your current weight, so something has to change. You're making a bit of an effort to eat well — you try to make sensible choices, you share your desserts — but it's time to kick it up a notch.

In the quiz above, check to see if you answered A to any of the questions. These are your weaknesses. Maybe it's the before-dinner bread basket that does you in. Maybe it's your inclination to eat everything on your plate. You need to buttress your weaknesses by having a plan. Set reasonable limits in advance and remind yourself of them just before you go into the restaurant. If you see your hand reaching for that bread basket, take that moment to pull it back and focus extra hard on the conversation at hand.

Now take a look at the C answer for every question. These are the answers of someone who is making a concerted effort to put reasonable amounts of healthy foods into her body. You need to move in this direction.

If your answers were mostly Cs:

Congratulations! You are making real choices about what and how much you want to eat. I applaud your efforts. Perhaps eating out isn't a problem for you. But if some of your answers were not Cs, look at them carefully. They will show you your weaknesses. You can eat plain chicken breast and salad until the cows come home, but it won't do you any good if you're following it up with a thick slab of chocolate-marshmallow-caramel mudslide or emptying a bottle or two of wine with every meal. Know your weaknesses. Isolate them, and work on them exclusively. You'll be surprised at what a difference one small, consistent change can make.

If your answers were mostly Ds:

Well, I have to give you kudos for your discipline. Rules are great, but you need to make sure they don't run your life. You run your life. Check in with yourself to make sure you're still enjoying yourself when you go out to eat. Maybe your rules are so habitual by now that you hardly notice them. But if you're constantly asking the waiter to put things on the side or to make substitutions, a little something is lost from the experience. Are you forcing the poor chef to replicate exactly what you eat at home? And if you're working so diligently to perfect your diet, why aren't you seeing results? Maybe it's time to stop looking at the food and look at the other facets of your life. Are you happy? Is this the life you want? Is this the home you want? Is this the body you want? Don't focus all your energy on minutia. Consider the big picture.

When and how much you eat

For some people, any step off your weekly food plan can be the first step down a slippery slope. You nibble one cookie and suddenly find yourself staring at an empty carton of ice cream and wondering how you managed to eat it without thinking. For others, a little break can fit in to your day or week without throwing your balance completely out of whack. You have to pay attention to yourself, maintain your food plan, and keep up with your journal and you will find what works for you.

Making sure that your kitchen and pantry and refrigerator are stocked only with those items that you know are good and healthy for you is a huge step. Removing temptation is another step. But when you leave the house, things become a little trickier. You know where your temptations lie. You know that a certain restaurant has a dessert you can't resist, or that every time you go to the movies you end up buying the large combo of drink, popcorn, and candy. Remember to keep your food journal so you can see clearly what made you stick to your plan and what made you slip. Don't just write down what you ate, but also how you felt and why you ate. Identifying those old patterns and habits will help you move forward. Only you can establish new patterns for the old ones. Be honest with yourself when you make the rules and when you break them until you find a solution.

Clutter is math. You can't have more books than you have bookshelf space. You can't eat cookies all day long and expect to feel good. Maybe you can't stand the sense of limitation and want to be able to pig out — to eat as many doughnuts as humanly possible. I can't show up on your doorstep to stop you from taking that route. You need to do it yourself. Don't leave yourself wiggle room. Be firm with yourself about quantity. Maybe you promise yourself you'll change the way you eat . . . tomorrow. Don't wait until after the weekend or until your schedule eases up.

This is your life. Don't put it on hold. Break the procrastination habit and get in the new habit of asking how the food you are reaching for fits in with what you want for yourself. Your body has its limits. Respect them.

Dear Peter:

One thing I always have to remind myself is I'm not getting a better value by clearing my plate. I like getting my money's worth so I like to finish my restaurant food, especially if it doesn't make a good leftover. But since I don't store fat for winter, I have to realize that eating more than my share isn't a good value. It's bad. Stomachaches, health problems, and weight changes aren't worth a "better value."

Make a commitment. Be sure that your plan involves less food and healthier food than what you currently eat. And don't change the rules. If you allow yourself that once-a-week doughnut, but a week later you find yourself munching on a whole plate, then clearly something is wrong. You aren't committed. (I'll talk more about cheating later in this chapter.)

Special Occasions and Holidays

Dear Peter:

We were invited to thirty-two graduation parties this year and attended as many as twelve in one day. These are invitations to weight disaster. Everyone puts out a huge spread of food and many will even tell you that it is bad luck not to eat a piece of their son's/daughter's graduation cake. It is terribly difficult to sit for hours on end, rambling down memory lane with friends who are all eating nonstop.

It's hard to say no to a birthday cake. It's someone's birthday! It only happens once a year! It's a special occasion! Same thing goes for pie on Thanksgiving. It's Thanksgiving! It's homemade pie! How can you say no? And when you go to a wedding, of course you raise a glass or two, or five. It's a once-in-a-lifetime event (one hopes). When you add them up, there sure are a lot of holidays and special occasions. This is a good thing — who doesn't love a party? — except when it comes to rich food and excessive drink.

Special occasions and holidays are everyone's favorite excuse for overeating. But a fun, festive life is full of such events, and we want your fun, festive life to be a long, healthy one. Just as you make rules for yourself concerning eating out, you need to plan for these special occasions. Take into account the particular temptations at holidays and celebrations. One of the simplest tricks is to eat well before you leave. Arriving full and satisfied instead of hungry helps you say no to that big slab of cake or groaning buffet table.

Hors d'oeuvres

A cheesy nibble here. A greasy taste there. They're so small. You're so hungry. Who can blame you? And who can keep track of how many they've had? They just keep coming and coming, and by the time it's all over you have no idea what you just ate. Watch out for hors d'oeuvres. Make rules and keep them. They're small but deadly.

Toasting

Many special events involve celebrating achievement or happiness with a lifted glass. Often a waiter comes around and refills that glass before you've even finished it. This is another situation where it's hard to keep track of how much you've had. Take small sips. Refuse refills until your glass is empty. Remember that no matter how easily it goes down, an alcoholic beverage is basically a dessert. Limit yourself. Too much booze can also cause brain fuzziness. You don't want to lose sight of the life you want to live (unless that life is a drunken haze). Rein in your drinks and you'll stay clear, live in the moment, and be able to remember all the fun you had when you wake up in the morning.

Traditions

Many celebrations, religious or otherwise, have rituals and traditions attached. Your mother-in-law's Christmas sugarplums. New Year's champagne. Chocolate on Valentine's Day. Beer and fried chicken on July Fourth. Never partake *just because* something is a tradition. Do it because it's meaningful to you, because you like the taste, because it's something you'll savor and remember, because you planned for it when you ate so carefully in the time leading up to this moment. Traditions are made to enhance moments, but they're no reason to set aside everything you've worked so hard for. You can participate without going overboard. Take a taste. Look around you. Absorb the essence of the moment and the reason for the tradition. Walk away with a sense of why you set aside time to gather with family or friends rather than with the sensation of a too-tight belt.

Peer pressure

"Go on — just one more bite, it's not going to kill you!" Peer pressure isn't just for teenagers. In every gathering lies a certain amount of social pressure, even if it isn't intentional or overt. You want to participate. You don't want to call attention to yourself. Anyone who has ever tried to abstain from drinking at a party knows that it's hard to go unnoticed. People think you're either pregnant or a reformed alcoholic. If you're either, chances are you're not dying to broadcast it to the whole party. Similarly, you may not want to spend a night out discussing your efforts to control your weight. Well, now is the time for you to get on your Mr. or Ms. Manners high horse. You have the right to make personal choices. And you have the right to ignore any raised eyebrows and to politely redirect any inappropriate questions. If someone says, "Not drinking tonight?" or "What? No dessert?? But you LOVE chocolate!" simply restate the obvious. Say, "No, thanks. It looks delicious, though." Then change the subject. Plan the diversion beforehand so that you're not caught unawares.

Buffets

Ah — the great American dream. The all-you-can-eat special that is just calling your name. Any all-you-can-eat buffet is the ultimate challenge for someone who is trying to control what they eat. Limitless food and limitless opportunity — what could be better? The rule for buffets is very simple: Take only one plate. Period. When you're encouraged to go back for seconds and thirds, even fourths, and you're given a clean plate each time, it's easy to lose track of how much you've had to eat. Imagine that the buffet is a menu, and decide what you want to order. Put a reasonable amount of these foods on your plate. Your plate shouldn't be overflowing with all different foods but should look like a simple, colorful, healthy plate of food. Eat slowly. Enjoy the conversation and the moment and the people you are with and tomorrow you won't regret having eaten, but instead will remember what a great time you had.

FOOD-CLUTTER PRINCIPLE

Focus on enjoying the next meal. Don't let one mistake make you give up.

CHEATING

Ten bucks says you've cheated on a diet. Who hasn't? Unless this is the very first time you've ever considered losing weight, you've cheated at some point. Because here you are, trying once again to lose that weight and get to that magic number on the scale that yells "Success!" But, remember, there's no diet in this book. This isn't a program with points and weigh-ins and a support group. Nobody is watching what you do. You are not on a diet. You are making a promise to yourself that you'll eat in a different way. You are moving from where you are to where you want to be. What's the point in lying to yourself? Keep in mind all of those things that the best you wants to do.

I was recently in New York speaking about my book *It's All Too Much*. A woman asked me how she could declutter her apartment. She responded enthusiastically to my suggestions until I said to her, "You have to stop buying anything new, except for essentials, for the next six months." Her mouth tightened into a straight-line smile and while she nodded yes, all I saw was no, no, no! When I pushed her on this point, she said that she was desperate to declutter her life and especially her living spaces, but to stop buying, no more shopping? She couldn't do that.

If you know anything about me you know that I can be a little tough at times. As harsh as it sounded, I told this woman that she wasn't serious about decluttering and there was nothing I could do for her. It may not have been what she wanted to hear, but it was definitely what she needed to be told. With food, as with clutter, there is no magic answer, no instant solution. I can show you what I have found to be the path to dealing successfully with the issue, but unless you're prepared to go wholeheartedly in that direction on your own, you may as well stop now. I can't do this for you, but you can absolutely do it yourself.

And so to cheating. Without honesty, there can be no success. You choose to cheat — it's as simple as that. When you cheat, the person you're shortchanging is yourself. It always fascinates me to meet people who hide the food they're eating. They eat at home where nobody can see them. Or they keep that one-pound bag of chocolate hidden in their desks so they can sneak out handfuls without anyone seeing. A client of mine lies in her Weight Watchers food diary. She says if she doesn't write that candy bar down it's like she never ate it. Who are you hiding from? The life you're sabotaging is your own.

Think about what you would do if you

watched a small child spill a glass of milk for the third day in a row. Would you tell her she was a horrible person? Would you say, "Oh, just give up. Go back to the bottle. You'll never be able to keep a glass of milk on the table." Of course not. You'd comfort her. You'd get her a fresh glass of milk. You'd talk to her about being aware of her body and being careful with glasses. And you'd encourage her to try again.

Slipups can be expected, since old habits are tough to change. It's important not to beat yourself up about that but rather to be gentle with yourself. Have faith. And start again. But don't forget self-examination. Children spill milk because they haven't learned self-awareness. They can't keep track of where their elbows are and joke with their friends at the same time. You're the adult here. Go back and look at your food journal. What tripped you up? Was it something that happened during the day? Were you busy and caught without a plan for a healthy meal? Did somebody say something to upset you? Remember your triggers? Go back and review them whenever you need some reinforcement. You need to face your triggers head-on. Change that part of your life or find a new outlet for that emotion. Work your triggers into your plan so they stop tripping you up when you least expect it.

Just because you cheat it doesn't mean you've failed. Don't let small mistakes snowball. See it for what it is (a doughnut, a double cheeseburger, a bag of potato chips), think about why it happened, and move on.

Remember your food journal

If you're struggling with external and emotional triggers, continue to use your food journal to identify the situations that lead you to bad food. Reviewing what you wrote will help you create substitute behaviors to overcome those weak moments.

Find healthy substitutions

Pick new behaviors to substitute for your external triggers. Mix and match from the examples below or make up your own.

INSTEAD OF:	I WILL:
Eating at cocktail parties . . .	Eat a healthy snack beforehand and allow myself a fixed number of hors d'oeuvres.

INSTEAD OF:	I WILL:
Having endless Friday drinks after work with colleagues . . .	Drink soda water with lemon or lime. No one needs to know what's in my glass.
Overindulging on Saturday nights eating out with friends . . .	Find healthy options on the menu and limit my portions.
Going crazy at holidays and special occasions . . .	Make rules: no birthday cake. Real dinners instead of party dinners.
Indulging when plans get canceled . . .	Have backup healthy food available at home.
Grabbing fast food . . .	Never grab anything. Plan.

INSTEAD OF EATING/DRINKING:	I WILL EAT:
Hors d'oeuvres	A piece of fruit and a handful of nuts
Nachos	Carrots and hummus
Cocktails	Soda water

For some people it's easier to substitute foods instead of behaviors. Try writing down your worst indulgences and picking healthy, filling alternatives or activities.

CHECKLIST
FOR CHAPTER NINE

- ☐ Identify the triggers that lead to overeating.
- ☐ Take the Know Your Weaknesses quiz.
- ☐ Know the events that lead to your overeating.
- ☐ Eliminate fast food.
- ☐ List ways to increase your level of physical activity.
- ☐ Maintain your food journal.
- ☐ Find healthy substitutions.

AFTERWORD:
THE SUCCESS YOU ENJOY

EMBRACING IT EVERY DAY

I speak all over the country about the work I do and the effect of clutter on people's lives. During the question-and-answer segment of every event, a hand inevitably goes up and somebody asks a question I hear over and over again: "You know all those families you work with, the ones we see on TV? Do they keep their places organized after you leave?" There is great fascination with whether it's possible for anyone to truly break their clutter habit and maintain their home.

While most people do achieve permanent change, I wish I could say that every family I work with is a success story, but that just isn't the case. However, over the years I have come to realize that there is a way of making the changes stick and making the new way of living a permanent one. Well, at least there's a way of greatly increasing the odds of being successful. Don't start with the "stuff," start with a clear idea of the life you want to be living. As for clutter, so for food: If you focus exclusively on the obvious (the stuff in your home or the stuff on your plate), you will never succeed in achieving any long-term success. The only way to stay on track is, oddly enough, to take a step back and ask yourself, What is it I want from my life? What life do I want to live? What does that life look like? This is a huge challenge and one that many people are too frightened to face. Fear of failure, and even fear of success and all its unanswered questions, has frequently stopped my clients from staying focused on their life goals. Ask the question. Follow the answer where it takes you.

No More Fat Butt

When you start to see changes, celebrate! Go out and eat whatever you want. Get a large fries and wash it down with a nice cold milkshake. Then grab another!

STOP! Sorry, I wasn't serious. If only it were that easy. I do want you to reward your progress, but don't do it by backsliding. Don't use food as a reward. Do something nice for yourself to celebrate your newly clutter-free butt. Let your success be a stepping-stone to other successes. Here are some suggestions:

- Give away the clothes that are too big for you.
- Go bathing suit shopping for the first time in years.
- Put together your own before and after photos. Put them on your mirror or someplace you'll see them every day and be reminded of how far you've come.
- Videotape yourself dancing naked.
- Take a dance class or try an activity you were always scared to do before.
- Splurge on a massage or spa weekend.
- Ask someone out on a date.

FOOD-CLUTTER PRINCIPLE

If you don't make mindful eating a way of life, the fat will creep back onto your butt.

THE JOY OF MAINTENANCE

What those fit and healthy people you see on the street don't tell you is that staying slender is much easier than losing weight. Think about it. To lose weight you need a deficit of calories — you have to burn off more than you take in. You need to use up more calories than you consume. That's hard. Your body knows it's getting a bum deal and lets you know loud and clear — it's hard to ignore the rumbling stomach or those pangs of hunger. But to maintain your weight, you just need to consume the same amount of calories that you burn. Much easier. Keep this in mind if you're not there yet. Losing weight is hard. Keeping it off is a little bit easier. There's light at the end of the tunnel.

The flip side to that is to remind yourself that you don't want to go through the tough weight-loss process again. Lock in the changes you've made by establishing a routine that doesn't make you feel deprived. Let yourself have treats, just make sure they are limited in two ways: frequency and quantity. You still have to make choices every day. If you start making choices that don't serve the life you wish to live, you'll find yourself right back where you started. There are a lot of delicious, fattening foods out there. Resisting them might be something you have to do whenever you're hungry, at every meal, for the rest of your life. Sounds daunting, but if the only other option is making bad choices that go against the life you want . . . well, it's your call.

Dear Peter:

My days often go through phases or cycles where things are out of control. I'm a single mom, a financial analyst, and writer who works out of my home with two autistic kids, so it's crucial that I keep things together and stay organized. With the craziness, I often fall short in this area. During those times when chaos is higher than normal, my home, or what I like to call my sanctuary, definitely shows it, and the clutter is embarrassing. I definitely also gain weight during those times. The frustration and overwhelming sense of failure when I look around not only causes me to turn to food for quick comfort, but the helplessness keeps me from exercising. This in turn causes more stress, I give up on trying to control things, and gain more weight. It's a horrible cycle. . . . The only way I have found to regain control during this spiral is to begin with the clutter — the rest inevitably follows.

Routine doesn't mean boring

You're starting to see changes because you've discovered a routine that works for you. You're eating less. You're eating foods that are better for you. Stick to it. But don't get in a rut. Life shouldn't be boring. The goal here isn't to live a dull, repetitive life with a skinny body. We've all met people who seem to be doing that and they don't seem like they're having much fun. After you're comfortable with your routine, but before you're bored, start to explore ways to expand your food horizons. Look for new recipes in magazines or cookbooks. Try entertaining — but this time instead of serving your friends food you know is drenched in butter, look for ways to serve tasty, healthy food. Crack open the grill, or make your first casserole. Buy an ethnic cookbook and explore new spices and cooking techniques. There are a million ways to be fun and adventurous without sacrificing any of what you've achieved.

Leave the fat behind behind

Healthy living should be a part of your life, but it shouldn't *be* your life.

- Don't define yourself by your relationship with food.
- Don't rob yourself of the joy of eating. If all your pleasure came from eating "bad" foods, find good foods or new interests to replace them. This is about

healthy, happy living — that's a goal worth striving for.

- Don't obsess. I care about you. I can't stand the idea of you turning into one of those people whose whole life is spent figuring out how not to eat a single potato chip.

- Don't count calories or eat fake foods or go to someone's house for dinner and tell them you brought your own meal.

- Don't pick the slivers of carrot out of your salad because someone told you carrots have lots of sugar.

- Don't share your opinions about what other people are eating. "Oh, I can't eat that — it's so fatty!" Be thoughtful and generous. Look for grace.

- Don't preach to your friends about how they can one day be as perfect as you. You really want to help someone? Feed the hungry, for heaven's sake!

Your ideal life and your ideal you

When I go into people's houses, either personally or through my books, and help them get rid of their clutter, I leave them with a clean house. With the stuff, it's easier in many ways because there you can see instant results. But, as I've said, there is no such thing as a quick fix. There is absolutely no guarantee that those decluttered homes will stay that way. Between junk mail and our consumer culture, they could be overwhelmed with stuff again in a matter of weeks. You have an even tougher road ahead. You can't follow the instructions in this book and lose all the weight in a week. Weight loss takes time; a healthy weight loss is one to two pounds a week — that's four pounds in a month, not the miracle forty pounds in thirty days that they advertise in the backs of magazines. Our bodies are much harder to declutter than our homes. That's why I want you to focus on being healthy, on achieving that list of activities that you want to be able to do with your ideal body. It's not about the scale. It's about your life.

Stick with it

Old habits die hard. As time passes, try to make more changes for the better. If you're happy about your weight, start thinking about your health. Are you eating heart-wise food? Are you exercising? Are you happy? Remember your goal. Remember your ideal life. You may make changes in leaps and spurts, as you find the time and energy; just remember that it's always within your power to control your life. You can create opportunities. Job opportunities come and go. Children grow up. New thoughts and ideas enter your mind. We are organisms. Our lives are organic. Let yours change, grow, and thrive. You'll feel young until you die.

ACKNOWLEDGMENTS

Writing this book has been a huge adventure — a little like the first Thanksgiving dinner I cooked a couple of years after I moved to America. There were about thirty-five people at that dinner and if I'd known the range of opinions on Thanksgiving cuisine — not to mention the recipe permutations — before I offered to host, maybe I'd have thought twice before offering to pull it all together. It's been a little bit the same with Does This Clutter Make My Butt Look Fat?

Growing up in a family of seven children, I don't recall my mother ever using any ingredients from cans or boxes to prepare meals. In retrospect, I have no idea how she did it. We were taught from a young age the importance of fresh food, well prepared. Meals were a central part of my childhood and even today, when my family gathers, it's generally about a table. It's loud and full of laughter, chaotic and crazy — I wouldn't

303

have it any other way. Food is central to the life of my family, as is a keen awareness that excess is seldom healthy.

In the same way that no meal makes itself, no book writes itself. And in the same way that there are a thousand variations on roasting a Thanksgiving turkey, there were a thousand — and more — opinions about clutter and fat. This book would not be in your hands if not for the help, humor, and insight of many people:

To the readers of the early manuscript: Holley Agulnek, Greg Batton, Lisa Giorgi-Poels, Andrew Mersmann, Dean Minerd, Andrea Rothschild-Feldman, and Cindy Seinar. These intrepid seven read and digested an early draft and returned with solid ideas and great suggestions. The book is stronger for their pages of feedback and focused insights.

To a wonderful wordsmith: Hilary Liftin. For making sure that I didn't choke on my own verbosity and for helping me shape the message, I owe her a huge debt for being there at every turn.

To the team at Free Press/Simon & Schuster: Jill Browning, Suzanne Donahue, Carisa Hays, Martha Levin, and Dominick Anfuso. Publisher, editor, publicist, advisor, critic, supporter, friend, business partner —

choose any of these, they all fit. An amazing team whose support and encouragement is enthusiastically given and gratefully received.

To a great agent: Lydia Wills and the team at Paradigm. There is no one who enjoys the giggle factor as much, nor anyone who keeps reminding me of the big picture quite so graphically. It's great to have her on my team — she knows how the game is played and lets me think an idea's mine even when we both know where it came from.

To my newest supporters: The team at Harpo Productions in Chicago. It's been a huge boost working with the teams from *The Oprah Winfrey Show,* the Oprah & Friends XM Radio group, and everyone behind Oprah.com. Their friendship, encouragement, and support have been invaluable — thanks to some of the most talented people in the business.

To the bravest of the brave: All the people who took the time to contact me with their thoughts and opinions about clutter and fat. Many of you will recognize yourself in these pages because without you, the book would have been impossible. I am constantly humbled by the generosity of people who share their stories and insights. I have received thousands of e-mails and each tells a tale that has affected the words on these pages. Thank you.

And to Ken — without whom none of this would be even remotely possible. But that's a whole new book!

When the meal is placed on the table, it's the chef who has the final responsibility for the flavors, the seasonings, and the taste. Even though there have been many cooks in the kitchen with this dish, I accept the final responsibility. Eat slowly. Enjoy.

INDEX

active lifestyle, 42, 43, 261–67
  examples of, 266–67
  exercise in, 77, 90, 101, 126,
      262–67
  television watching vs., 101
advertising, impact on overeating, 56
alcohol, as external temptation, 271, 276,
      280, 281, 282
aspirational foods, 175

balance:
  client letters about, 260–61
  of lifestyle, 188, 260
  meals and, 209–11, 228
  bathroom, 80, 139, 145
  bedroom, 138, 145
  clutter in, 21
  purposes of, 21, 136, 145
body:
  change in, 48, 51, 79, 90, 92–93
  client letters about, 89–90, 132–33

and risks associated with being fat, 35,
   41, 48, 51, 59, 61–62
Healthier Choices Chart, 193, 194, 197,
   198
hiking, 265
holidays, *see* special occasions
home, 131, 133, 134
   chaos and, 74, 75, 135
   client letters about, 195, 220
   happiness and, 19
   room-by-room tour of, 136–42
hors d'oeuvres, 270, 281

ice-skating, 265
ideal weight, 90
immediate gratification, culture of, 13–14,
   24, 223
   debt in, 13
It's All Too Much (Walsh), 15, 34–35, 66,
   131, 132, 137, 285
   client letters about, 26–28, 29–30, 131,
   133, 148

job:
   satisfaction with, 44–45, 46, 184
   weight discrimination at, 59
journal, food, 118, 216, 277, 287, 288
   junk food, 123, 124, 128, 190, 202, 212,
   228, 237
   as cause of weight gain, 56, 144

organization (*continued*)
  of recipes, 172
  of refrigerator, 167–70, 277
  overeating, 258–59
  advertising's impact on, 56
  client letters about, 26–28, 117, 132–33,
    279
  reasons for, 75–76, 280
  as result of more-for-your-money princi-
    ple, 279
  see also portion size; temptations, exter-
    nal
overweight, *see* fat, overweight

pantry, 172–80
  and avoiding external temptations, 277
  clean-out of, 74, 173–74
  client letters about, 173
  list of unnecessary foods in, 175–78
  organization of, 178–80
  planning for, 173–74
  purpose of, 172
  shopping for, 173–74
peer pressure, 283
planning:
  absence of, 147, 237, 238
  client letters about, 271
  daily, 182–83
  food and, 75, 76, 123, 144, 167–70, 185,
    195–205, 241

ABOUT THE AUTHOR

Part contractor, part therapist, **Peter Walsh** lives to conquer clutter and help people re-organize their personal spaces. As the organizational guru on TLC's hit show *Clean Sweep,* a regular guest on *The Oprah Winfrey Show,* and the voice of reason on his weekly national radio program, *The Peter Walsh Show,* Peter demonstrates that decluttering is the sure path to a richer, fuller life.

Peter holds a master's degree with a specialty in educational psychology, has worked internationally in corporate training and health promotion, and possesses a keen sense of humor that regularly gets him out of the toughest situations. When not leading those lost in clutter to a happier, less-stressed life, Peter divides his time between Los Angeles and Melbourne, Australia.

The employees of Thorndike Press hope you have enjoyed this Large Print book. All our Thorndike and Wheeler Large Print titles are designed for easy reading, and all our books are made to last. Other Thorndike Press Large Print books are available at your library, through selected bookstores, or directly from us.

For information about titles, please call:
(800) 223-1244

or visit our Web site at:
http://gale.cengage.com/thorndike

To share your comments, please write:
Publisher
Thorndike Press
295 Kennedy Memorial Drive
Waterville, ME 04901